the *Christian*
Herb Gardener's Handbook

A Beginner's Guide

the *Christian*
Herb Gardener's Handbook
A Beginner's Guide

Meg Grimm

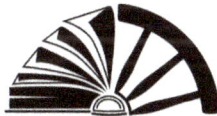

Story Spinner Press

www.storyspinnerbooks.com

Published by
Story Spinner Press
Ohiopyle, Pennsylvania
www.storyspinnerbooks.com

All Scripture quotations, unless otherwise indicated, are taken from THE HOLY BIBLE, NEW INTERNATIONAL VERSION®, NIV® Copyright © 1973, 1978, 1984, 2011 by Biblica, Inc.® Used by permission. All rights reserved worldwide.

The website addresses and print books recommended throughout this book are offered as resources and do not in any way imply an endorsement on the part of Story Spinner Press.

This book contains information relating to the use of herbs. It is designed for your personal knowledge and to help you be a more informed consumer. It is not intended to replace medical advice from your physician. No expressed or implied guarantee of the effects of the use of the recommendations can be given or liability taken. The materials in this book are not meant to take the place of diagnosis and treatment by a qualified medical practitioner or therapist.

First Printing, April 2020

Printed in the United States of America

ISBN 978-1-7347867-0-5

Library of Congress Control Number: 2020905553

This little book is dedicated to my husband Max.
You make all my dreams come true.

Contents

Equipped for the Journey

The Herb Garden

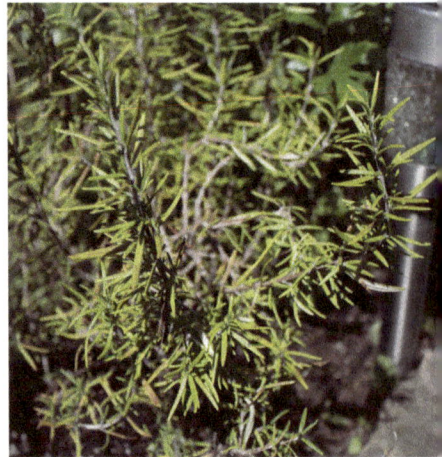

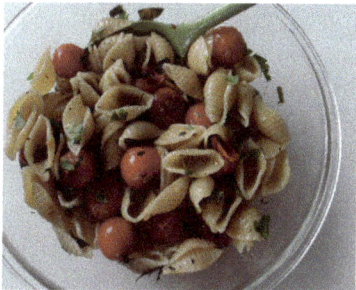

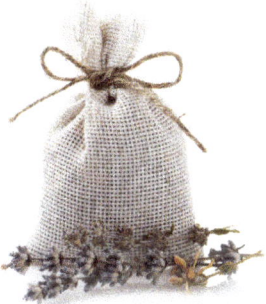

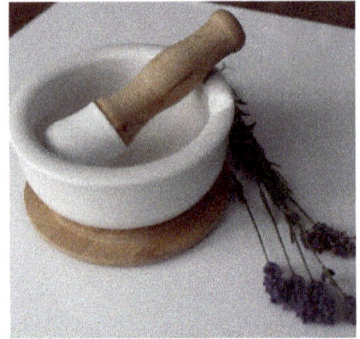

Herbs and Oils of the Bible

Relevant Herbs at a Glance

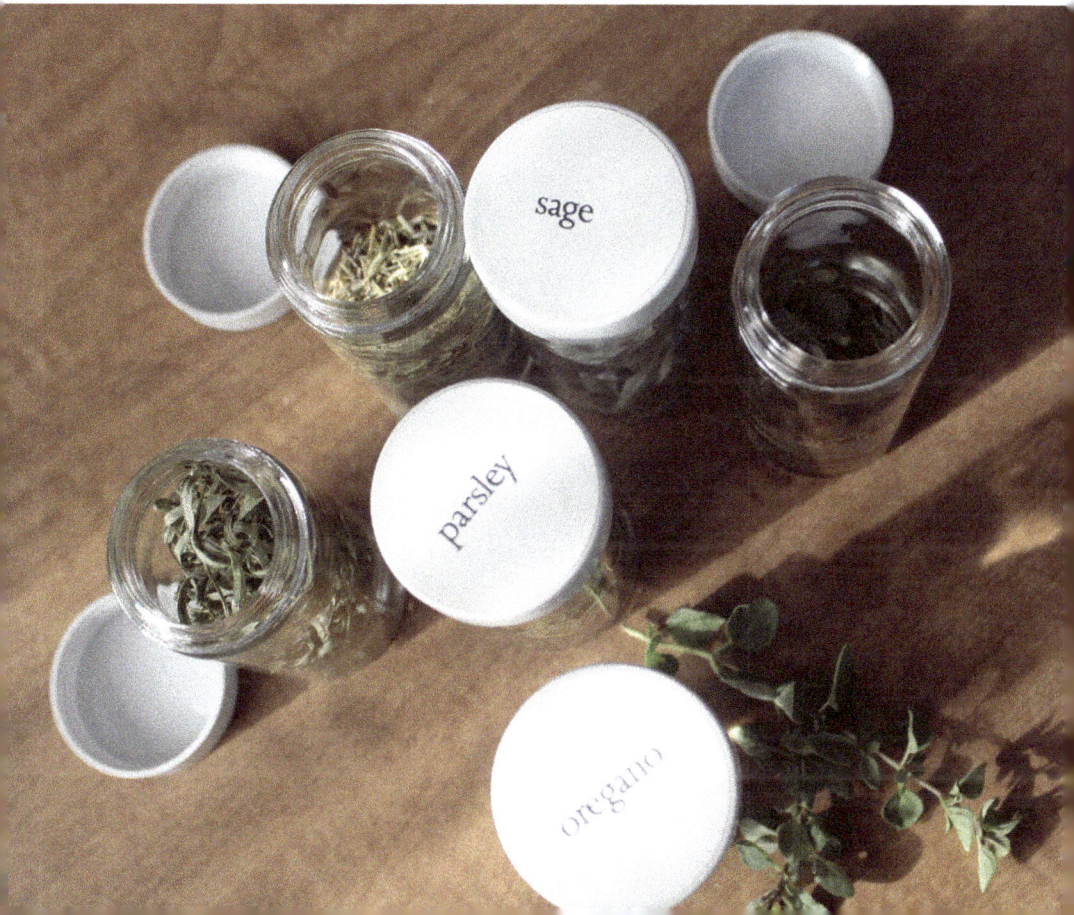

Dear Reader,

For me, it began with a love for history. I wanted to know how people cared for their bodies in Bible times. I wanted to prepare medicines the same way a medieval healer might. I wanted to walk through the forest with my apron or basket like a peasant of old knowing what all the plants were and how they could be used.

When I first started to grow my own herbs, I was thrilled to discover how easy it was to work with them. Regrettably, experimenting became so exciting that I did not notice an unwelcome visitor who had joined me on my adventure until it was almost too late.

It was not the first time evil had subtly lured me closer to itself by way of herbs. Years ago, one of my favorite movies had been "Practical Magic." Before that, as a twelve-year-old, I had also fallen victim to a brief interest in witchcraft when "The Craft" was released. The notion of herbal healing had always enchanted me. Though now I was a Christian adult who thought I understood the difference between witchcraft and gardening, the boundaries were more shrouded than I could have imagined.

Of course, herbs are not evil. Growing and harvesting them is sensible, and I encourage it. Cooking with herbs and creating herbal products for body care is not unwise.

A problem arises when the occult infiltrates Christian thought, Christian churches, and of course, Christians themselves. This may not seem likely or frequent, but then there would be no purpose for this book. With complementary and alternative medicine on the rise today, energy-based concepts of the occult have been re-packaged as God-gifted healthcare. The tactic is particularly designed to trick and trap faithful men and women of God. The realm of plant medicine and its subfields are espcially growing in popularity today. There is much for Christians to be watchful about, from erroneous folklore to deceptive marketing.

I created this book to illuminate the boundaries of herbal usage otherwise blurred by shadows. If you are a Christian interested in cultivating your own herb garden and putting the plants to use, this book will help you navigate that journey with discernment and vigilance.

May the tools of these pages be a blessing to you and those whose lives you touch.

Peace to you in Christ Jesus,

Meg Grimm

Equipped *for the* Journey

Before exploring herbs, the first three sections of this book will provide the tools needed to avoid spiritual pitfalls and physical dangers on the path.

*See to it that no one takes you captive through hollow
and deceptive philosophy, which depends on human
tradition and the elemental spiritual forces of this world
rather than on Christ. Col. 2:8*

Discerning the Anti-Christian Philosophies of Herbalism

For many Christians, an interest in healing properties of herbs first came from disenchantment with conventional medicine. Whether or not the reasons were justified, conventional medicine was deemed cold, out of reach, unaffordable or untrustworthy.

Of course, nonbelievers are attracted to natural means of healing, too. But since Christians can view herbal healing as alignment with God's original intention for healthcare, they may be susceptible to spiritual deceptions of herbalism in other ways. An innocent desire to understand plants in order to be closer to our Creator can become a gateway into accepting occult-based therapies of alternative medicine.

Before we go any further, let's talk about terminology.

The term *herbalism* is often associated with a pantheistic worldview, viewing the use of herbal remedies as part of humanity's oneness with nature. It is a religious approach. On the other hand, the term *herbal medicine* refers to using herbal remedies as chemicals with physical effects. (18:203) This distinction is rarely made, and the terms are often used interchangeably. Since there is indeed a difference between the two concepts, I make the distinction in this book using that terminology.

Let's now explore where herbal medicine ends and herbalism begins.

At first, the idea that herbs have an advantage over pharmaceuticals is easy to accept. Pharmaceutical drugs contain a single active substance while herbs provide an array of catalysts working together. Drugs are synthetic. Herbs are used in their natural form. Drugs produce side effects. Herbs do not quickly build up in the body.

So far, so good, right? Who would not want to give herbs a try?

The trouble with the thought process may have already begun, however. An herbalist's view for herb superiority has to do with the self-healing capacity of the body. Herbalists tend to believe that herbs activate this power.

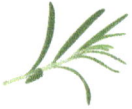

> An herbalist is described as one who deals in herbs, especially medicinal herbs.

While there may be a pharmacological action (chemical action) of herbs on the body to promote the healing claims, the dominant feature ascribed to herbs by many herbalists is not in the realm of supported science. From this point, herbalism becomes another arena altogether. Perhaps considered more important than pharmacology, another component of herbal action is understood to be *energy*.

In general, the key concept of most alternative medicine is that energy in the body must be flowing correctly for optimal health. A term gaining popularity today is **energy medicine**. Energy medicine is an umbrella term encompassing numerous therapies from all over the world. A practitioner's role is not to attack disease but to maintain natural energy flow – to regain balance in the body. To them, when one experiences symptoms, it is an indication of an underlying energetic imbalance. Within herbalism, the healing properties, or "energies" of herbs, are matched with symptoms, root causes and diseases. (8) Recommended herbs are said to restore balance, thus correcting root problems. As a result, symptoms are meant to go away.

It is important to note that the energy model redefines disease as it is known in Western medicine. It is foreign to the conventional approach. Energy medicine is also not supported by science. Yet, if one does accept that humans are conduits of energy and all disease is energy-based, the foundation has been laid to embrace a belief system contrary to the Christian faith.

In fact, many alternative medicine therapies in use today are no different from occult magic. All manner of occultists use the same energy as that of energy medicine practitioners in order to achieve their desires. (1:74-75) Healing is only one desired outcome in magical practice, but it may be the beginning of embracing manipulation of energy for other sorcery and witchcraft. (8)

> **Whether European, Native American, Chinese, Western, Ayurvedic, or any other herbal medicine system, the common thread among them all is the concept of plant energy working in synergy with the natural energy of individuals. (8)**

The following allegory was once suggested by a Christian pharmacist. Imagine a tree. The leaves of the tree represent energy-based medicine practices, such as herbalism. The branches of the tree are the false philosophical systems, such as the New Age religious thought systems. The trunk is occult practice, and the root is satanic deception. (8)

Let's talk about words again.

The word *balance* is not inherently a bad word. Neither is *harmony*, *energy*, or *spiritual*. Therefore, Christians may not experience red flags when hearing language like this. They might accept and adapt the rhetoric themselves. They might assume, like I did, that an imbalance in the body refers to a nutrient deficiency that can be brought back into balance by consuming certain plants and herbs. However, the language of herbalism pre-conditions even Bible-believing Christians to accept other concepts of energy medicine.

The process goes something like this.

Someone may accept that human beings have an energetic life force flowing through their bodies. They are told that the same energy flows through everything else in the universe.

Next, they may come to believe that since this universal life force flows through everything, it also *connects* them with everything. Good or bad energy from others can even affect their own health. Consequently, this person may feel empowered to use the special energy for their benefit and the benefit of others. They believe disease can be avoided by maintaining the body's balance using simple techniques. The power has always been within them, whether or not science has yet understood it.

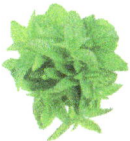

> **Some practitioners of alternative medicine therapies even claim to heal clients from across great distances using an energetic connection.**

At the same time, a person on this journey is typically being persuaded to distrust conventional medicine. Consider a 2018 advertisement from The HeartMath Institute for The Energy Medicine & Healing Summit. It promises the ability to unlock inner power and "take health into your own hands." It reads: "While traditional western medicine focuses on diagnosing symptoms and treating you from the outside, energy medicine unlocks your life force to heal you from the inside – and addresses the root causes of illness. You can tap into your own inner resources to treat ailments, increase vitality and help prevent disease."

Finally, this person may easily arrive at the conclusion that God must be the special life force. If God is in everything, everything is in God. Or, the more accurate wording of the deception is that *God is everything, and everything is God*. In the end, *we are God*. This is the pantheistic New Age movement, the foundation of which is the occult.

Many Christian practitioners of alternative medicine therapies do not take the final plunge into believing *God is everything, and everything is God*. Yet they have still been deceived into believing they are accessing universal energy to promote healing. For many herbalists, energy within herbs balances the energy of the body.

But what, or who, is the real source behind this supposed power?

Matthew 24:24 warns, "For false messiahs and false prophets will appear and perform great signs and wonders to deceive, if possible, even the elect."

Paul also tells Timothy, "The Spirit clearly warns that in later times some will abandon the faith and follow deceiving spirits and things taught by demons. (1 Tim. 4:1)

It feels contrary to our doctrine to believe that healing could ever come from the occult. However, we also know that Satan masquerades as an angel of light. (2 Cor. 11:14) Scripture warns of demonic counterfeits being used to deceive. Therefore, healing miracles that we may witness or experience from energy medicine are not what we think. They are enticing hooks meant to pull victims down a dangerous path. Would you want to take a concoction of herbs that has been enchanted by a witch who consulted her familiar spirit for the recipe, even if it "works?" When worded like that, a Christian would readily decline. However, sometimes the ways in which we participate in using herbs are no different. The truth is simply veiled. Beware! Even if an herbalist is a Christian, there is no guarantee they are not deceived.

Although a Christian can learn to use herbs to promote healing bio-chemically without falling prey to anti-biblical philosophies, danger will always be lurking in the field. Speech used across alternative medicine subtly leads others toward pantheistic ideas rather than truths of God. Often, mentions of God become part of the deception.

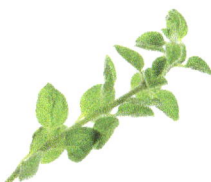

I once began coursework to obtain a board-certification as a Complementary and Alternative Healthcare Practitioner. I walked away from the endeavor when I discovered occult roots in several of the techniques of the field. During my years of involvement with these areas of alternative medicine, I regularly heard and spoke the language. The following are examples of deceptive speech that I will share from my experiences.

"They (herbs) are characterized by an energetic nature manifested through a complex set of molecules evolved to adapt to the environments in which they live… We need them much more than they need us. Greet them with gratitude and respect and they will serve you well… Your herbal allies will truly become your teachers." – Professor Scott Stuart in a lecture, "Safety and Dosage Guidelines in Herbal Medicine," from the American College of Healthcare Sciences.

"In our fast-paced culture, we're becoming increasingly disconnected from nature, and in doing so, we're losing touch with our symbiotic relationship with the plant kingdom…a vast life-giving resource for healing our bodies, balancing our emotions, and awakening our consciousness." – The Shift Network, email advertisement for the Plant Medicine Summit in 2019.

"Plant and herb essences are like the personality, or spirit, of the plant." – Robert Tisserand, known as the world's leading expert in Aromatherapy, in his book *The Art of Aromatherapy: The Healing and Beautifying Properties of the Essential Oils of Flowers and Herbs.* (1:259)

Even The Herbal Academy: International School of Herbal Arts and Sciences, an online site that provides herbal studies programs focused on evidence-based herbalism only, still publishes articles containing spiritual practices and ideas. There are references to reiki, chakras, flower essences and more on their blog and in other teaching material.

As an example, in an educational article in the Herbal Academy's subscription database titled "Bringing the Thyroid into Balance Naturally," a writer describes using flower essences: "If the hyperthyroid disease was preceded by an intense stressful event, I would also incorporate a few drops of flower essences specific to the individual's patterns and situation into the herbal tincture blend. Potential flower essences include bleeding heart (letting go), comfrey (deep healing), Echinacea (foundational healing), honeysuckle (moving on), or lavender (spirit calm)."

Anti-Christian philosophies are such an integral part of herbalism that unsullied herbal medicine is difficult to find. In lectures or in literature about herbalism, experts in the field may begin with compelling scientific information, but they so often lead to the spiritual realm.

The following is a generalized example of the progression that I have assembled based on my previous exposure.

"Specific berries and seeds support the health of your nervous system, liver, kidneys and immunities," begins the speaker.

The lecturer may then go on to promise mental and emotional health: "They enhance memory and mental clarity…"

Since some herbs have been shown to calm the nerves or help with depression, this may still sound acceptable.

Then it happens.

"…and inner harmony."

The leap from potential pharmacological benefits to spiritual ones has now been made. By the end of the lecture, the speaker may recommend a meditation for meeting the spirit of a plant "whose berries and seeds are used for these purposes."

If you do not catch the subtle switches that are universally laced throughout the language of herbalism, the statements may start to sound possible, and then normal, and then exciting. That is how deception works.

Sometimes, language is not so obvious. It is best to check the credentials of a practitioner to discover if they are aligned with other practices of energy medicine, such as reiki, reflexology, acupuncture and yoga. That is a clue to be on guard.

However, if the problem is with language, we can understand that plants contain no mystical power themselves. They are merely implements behind which spirit powers can work, not unlike crystals, tarot cards, pendulums, dowsing rods and other tools used by the occult. However, keep in mind that the occult has specifically utilized herbs and plants for centuries. Plants are often said to possess human attributes, even having a personality. They are believed to have etheric spiritual essences sometimes referred to as souls. The essence of the plant is said to work powerfully upon the mind and emotions.

In the New Testament, the Greek word *pharmakeía* is translated as "sorcery" or "witchcraft." From this word, we derive our word "pharmacy." The connection between medicine and magic within an occult framework is clear. It is one reason why God commanded His people to be separate from the practices of the cultures that surrounded them.

In addition, many herbalists also use occult methods for diagnosis and determining treatments, such as muscle testing (Applied Kinesiology) or a pendulum, further linking herbalism with the energies of the occult. Cooperating with this energy is said to not only produce health but also connect users with nature – more specifically, "divine, cosmic forces of the universe."

Rituals are also often implemented into practices of herbalism. During my time in the field, I would often come across odd instructions, such as, "Bring the teapot to the prepared water, not the water to the teapot," or, "Approach the client on his right side, not his left." In incidents like these, it is usually assumed that there is some evidence-based reason. Therefore, many of these occult-rooted rituals are not questioned. For me, the more deceived I became, the less I questioned the questionable.

Finally, when using herbs for healthcare purposes, a Christian must not only be vigilant of spiritual dangers for their own protection, but they should also consider their influence on others. (1 Thess. 5:22) It is essential to clarify that techniques being used are based on the pharmacological actions of the herbs, not their energies. Do not be afraid to warn others of occult dangers. (Eph. 5:8-11) In addition, efforts should be made to not use the New Age language of some herbalists and other alternative medicine practitioners. The threat of New Age in medicine is real, and it is found in many Christian churches.

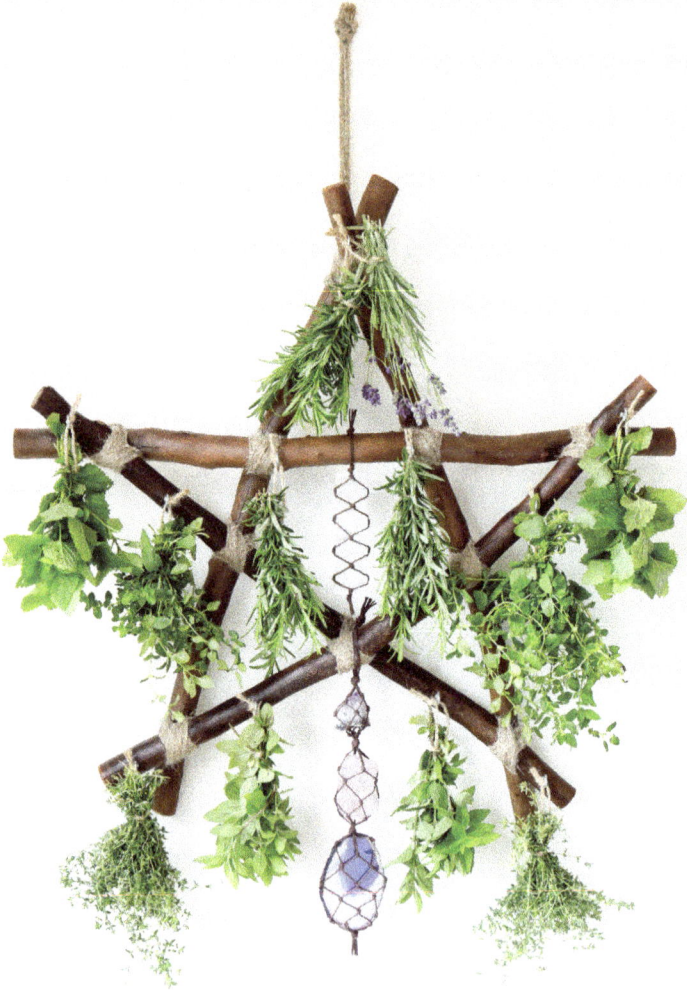

Throughout history, herbs, plants and their "etheric energies" have been used for diagnosis, healing, psychic development and altered states of consciousness. In ancient times, medicine and religion were part of the same discipline, and magic was most often a department. (11:4) Only in the Hebrew culture is this model not authenticated. (20:14)

Hallucinogenic herbs and other preparations are still used today in witchcraft and shamanism to access the spirit world. (18:204) No matter what pretty packaging may cover these occult practices today, it is still practicing magic. The Bible calls this divination, witchcraft and sorcery. (Deut. 18:9-13)

If your personal use of plant remedies may send confusing messages to other Christians, leave medicinal usage of herbs to the occultists. (Rom. 14:13-23) You may not be deceived yourself, but someone else could fall victim. Since the world uses language tied to pantheistic philosophies when speaking about plant medicine, others will inevitably be exposed to it. In fact, most Christians who have fallen victim to occult bondage from an alternative medicine therapy say they initially trusted it because another Christian did.

If you have become involved in energy medicine practices, understand that our enemy is crafty and seeks only to steal, kill and destroy. (John 10:10) Repent now! (1 John 1:9) Follow the example of Acts 19:18-19:

Many of those who believed now came and openly confessed what they had done. A number who had practiced sorcery brought their scrolls together and burned them publicly. When they calculated the value of the scrolls, the total came to fifty thousand drachmas.

The Bible continually warns against looking to or worshipping created things rather than the Creator. (Rom. 1:25) This is idolatry. The wonderful, simple, bondage-breaking truth is that *Jesus is our Healer*. (Exod. 15:26)

Potential Dangers of Herbal Medicine to the Body

Anti-Christian philosophies are not the only threat lurking undetected in the realm of plant medicine. Since herbal remedies are widely accepted as natural and safe, very real physical dangers are often unperceived.

Minimal Credible Information

Despite the advocacy literature abounding today, it is important to know that there are limited valid medical studies on herbs used for medicine – on their safety, effectiveness or mechanisms of action. Some of the more serious adverse reactions of certain plant species have not been recognized until recently, such as kidney failure, cancer, respiratory problems and liver damage. Furthermore, little is known about the amount of an herbal remedy that can be considered a safe dose for an adult. The authors of *Alternative Medicine: The Christian Handbook* recommend that adults should limit intake to short periods of time unless long-term studies have been conducted. Children should not take herbal remedies at all unless proven safe. (18:203)

Delayed Treatment

As John Ankerberg and John Weldon note in their book *Can You Trust Your Doctor*, many users of herbal remedies choose to not tell their doctors. Whether they are concerned that the practice will be frowned upon or they simply believe the natural products are safe, herbal remedies can interfere with a doctor's recommendations or a patient's prescriptions. Meanwhile, if the herbal remedy is an ineffective alternative treatment but is being used exclusively, it will delay or prevent appropriate treatment. In this way, a serious illness may progress. (1:254)

Ignorance

The most common assumption about herbal remedies is that they are not drugs. They are. They are natural chemicals with the potential to cause harm, and they can certainly interact adversely with other medications. Since herbal medicine is widely unregulated and information is limited, it is impossible to know how much herbal remedies have contributed to illness and death through the years. (4)

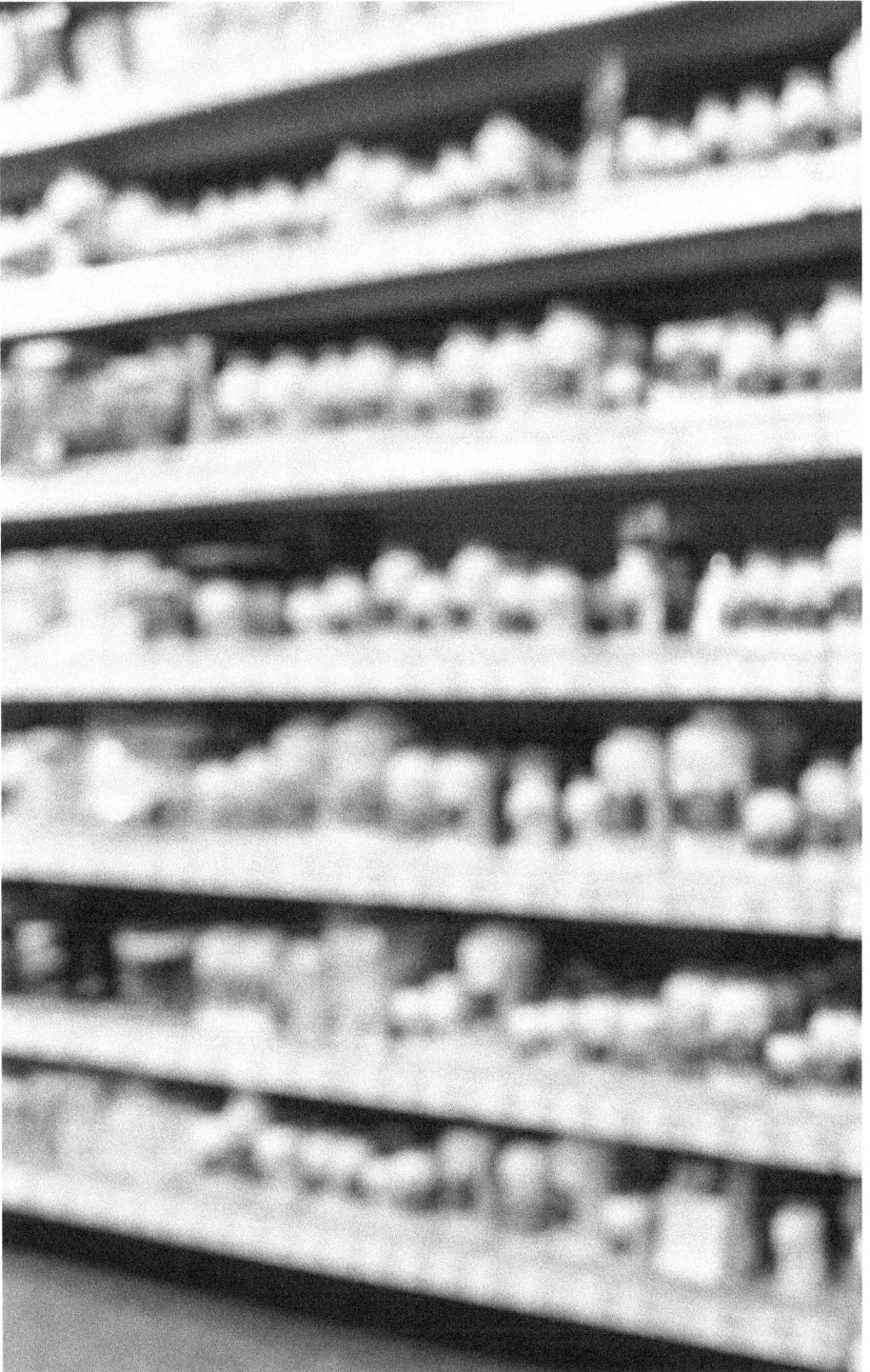

Deceptive Supplement Industry

Let no one deceive you with empty words, for because of such things God's wrath comes on those who are disobedient. Therefore do not be partners with them. Eph. 5:6-7

When not harvesting the plants on their own, consumers may not know if the herbal supplements they purchase on the market contain what the label suggests. Testing of DNA has shown that many pills labeled as healing herbs are little more than powdered rice and weeds, or worse.

A study published in the journal *BMC Medicine* in 2013 found that a product advertised as black cohosh – a North American plant popular for helping with hot flashes and other menopause symptoms – instead contained an Asian plant that can be toxic to humans. Many other studies in recent years have suggested a sizable percentage of herbal products are not what they claim to be. (13,17)

Contributing to the issue is that consumers often consider herbal supplements safe until proven guilty; unlike the scrutiny they place on prescription drugs. Instead, health is entrusted to an industry with so few safeguards that, according to the study, an estimated 33 percent of products on the market are adulterated, contaminated or mislabeled.

A paper by forensic pathologist Roger Byard published in 2010 in the US-based *Journal of Forensic Sciences* analyzed the toxic substances found in many herbal products.

Byard writes, "As access to such products is largely unrestricted...their contribution to death may not be fully appreciated during a standard autopsy...Forensic pathologists the world over need to become more aware of the contribution that herbal medicines are playing in a range of deaths that is not currently recognized." (25)

Despite the issue, Grandview Research, Inc. reported in 2018 that the global herbal supplements market size is expected to reach USD 8.5 billion by 2025.

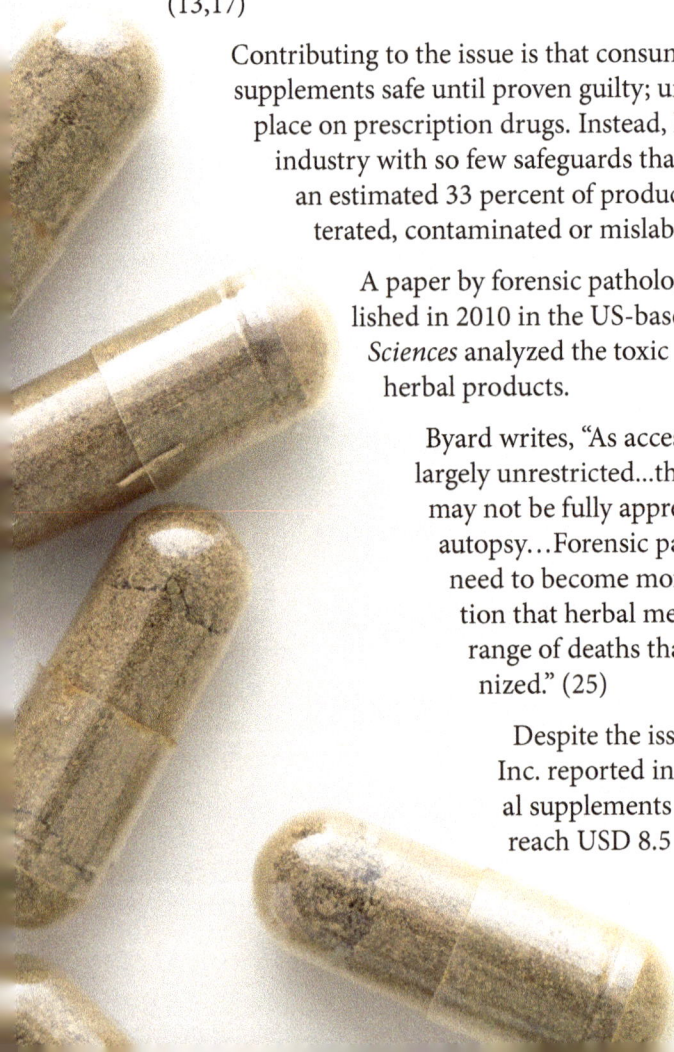

If you are an herbal supplement user, you may be familiar with the onset of unfavorable symptoms, such as headaches, when starting new supplements. Alternative medicine practitioners explain that the products cause the body to detox. Clients need only drink plenty of water and not be concerned.

However, consider that the same 2013 study showed that one bottle labeled St. John's wort contained only Alexandrian senna, an Egyptian yellow shrub that is a powerful laxative. Some Gingko biloba supplements were also tested with DNA barcoding to reveal they contained nothing more than fillers and black walnut. (13,17) Therefore, adverse symptoms may be caused by something other than a detox. Those with allergies may be especially at risk.

All in all, the supplement industry is filled with questionable practices. It may be better to harvest the plants on your own if possible. Always check with your doctor for recommendations, and research supplement companies before purchasing.

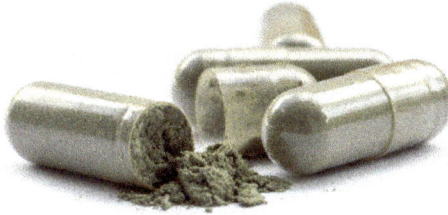

Unlike pharmaceuticals, herbal supplements are not studied rigorously using randomized, controlled clinical trials. Serious and even fatal interactions have been reported. In fact, Cleveland Clinic cardiologists warn that anyone who takes cardiac medicines should not use supplements at all without first checking with their doctor. (9)

How to Use Herbs Safely

*The wisdom of the prudent is to give thought to their
ways, but the folly of fools is deception. Prov. 14:8*

Occult-based herbalism is separate from the scientific study of the health properties of herbs, though the distinction is sometimes difficult to decipher by the laymen. Pharmacognosy, pharmacology and other related disciplines require biology and chemistry. Whereas the New Age approach to herbalism can be described as a commercial enterprise. Dr. Varro Tyler, previously one of the nation's foremost experts on herbal medicine, once branded herbalism as being comprised of outdated information, folklore, superstition, wishful thinking and even hoax. Today, mystical and miraculous claims are still made in the field. Diabetes cannot be cured by pumpkin seeds or black walnuts, for instance. (1:252)

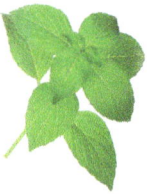

> There is a lack of uniformity for treatment across the field of herbalism. An herbalist may prescribe almost any herbal remedy for any given symptom. (1:255)

The best way to use herbs as medicine is to treat them with the same respect as conventional drugs. Some herbs are inherently toxic. Many have side effects. All should be used with intelligence and understanding.

Although it is true that herbal remedies are milder and less concentrated than pharmaceuticals, the following safety measures should be practiced when using herbs as medicine.

Personal Confidence

One should have personal confidence in the properties and effects of an herb or plant.

To begin with, spend some time researching the plant to be used. According to information derived from the American College of Healthcare Sciences, herbs are categorized as mild, medium or toxic. Mild herbs are generally considered safe, such as thyme, garlic, basil and lavender. Medium herbs, such as peppermint, juniper berry, sage and valerian, should only be used for a short duration. They have potential for toxic accumulation. Toxic herbs, such as foxglove and nightshade, should never be used at all.

In addition, keep in mind that if you are allergic to one herb in a botanical family, you are likely allergic to the others.

Next, be sure that the person supplying an herbal treatment or providing information is qualified. Personally, I check to see if they are associated with energy medicine practices. I use more caution if an author's qualifications include titles like "board-certified doctor of natural medicine," "licensed acupuncturist," "skills in flower essences," "energy healer," "spiritual teacher" and so on.

Note: It is rare that I find an expert in the field of herbal healing who is not associated with energy medicine in some way. Information from these sources can seem science-based at first, but before long, the speaker or writer inevitably indicates underlying anti-Christian philosophical views. At that point, it is unclear if the remainder of their information is trustworthy. However, sometimes information needed may not be contingent on the source's philosophical background. Wise discernment is essential.

Third, be sure that scientific testing has established effectiveness and provided information about potential side effects or allergic reactions for the herb in question.

Finally, if using an herbal supplement on the market, be confident that the labeling is correct and no contamination exists. (See ***Credible Sources***.)

If you are not confident in all of these areas, it may be best to not take the risk.

Credible Sources

A credible source means it is unbiased and supported with evidence. Was it published on a reputable, non-biased web site? Or in a scholarly journal? Is it an in-depth study complete with an abstract, reference list and documented data? What are the credentials of the writers? Are they respected and well-known? Even so, in what field are they well-known? Many experts of alternative therapies are practicing energy medicine. A Christian should be cautious about information accepted from such a source.

The databases on page 17 contain known information about herbs that has been proven with controlled studies. If what you hear about a certain herb is not listed, it may not be true. In the end, tradition and folklore are still sources for some of the so-called known information about herbs. When supposed scientific study is briefly mentioned, it is best to double-check. Are there multiple credible sources? That is even better.

Some proponents of herbal medicine believe that if an herbal remedy is found ineffective in testing, the problem is with the test. It is impossible to prove otherwise since no further testing has been conducted. However, it is better to trust what is known rather than what is not.

Another helpful safeguard is the United States Pharmacopeia (USP) stamp of approval. The USP is a national group that evaluates the standards for which drugs and herbal medicines are manufactured. Subscribe to ***www.consumerlab.com*** to find out if an herbal remedy brand has been tested by the USP.

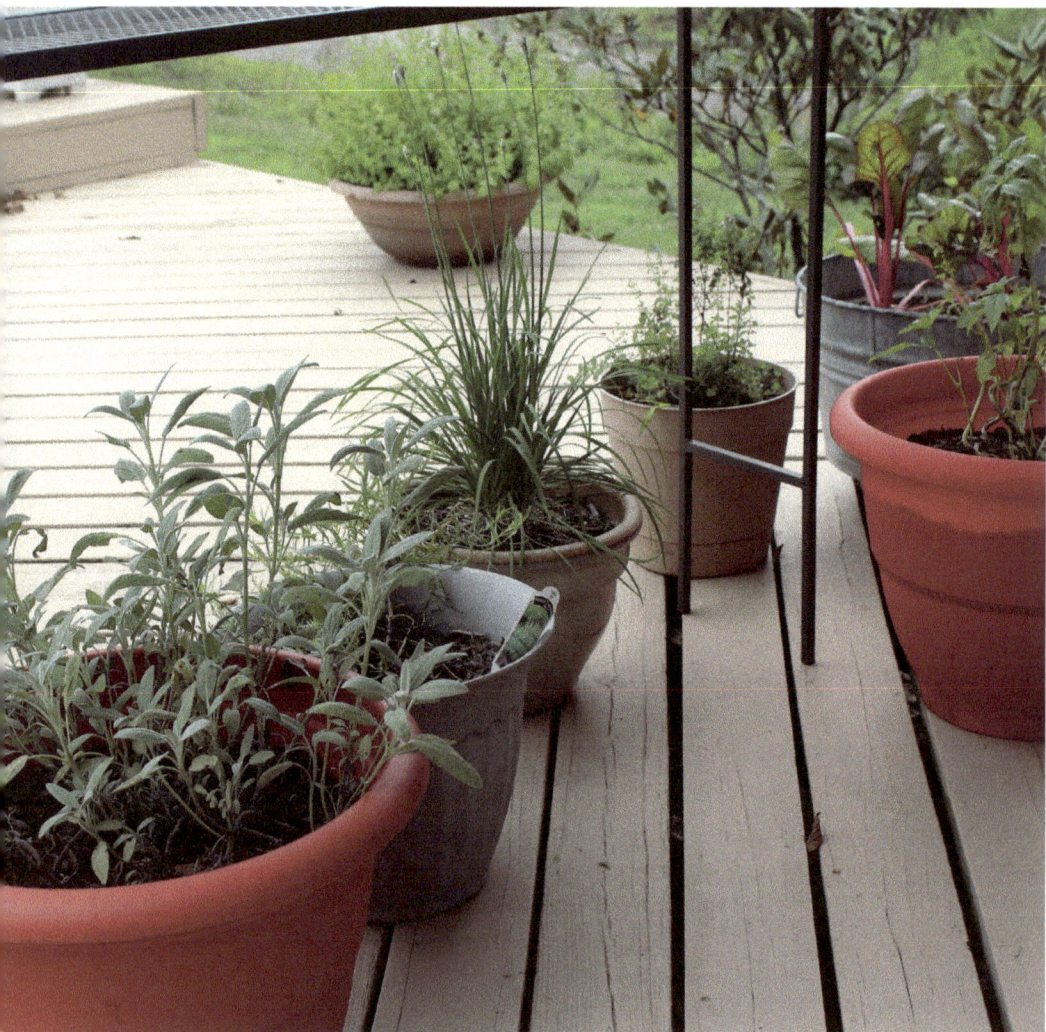

Herbal Monographs

A monograph provides an organized set of information on a subject compiled into a report. An herbal monograph, specifically, gives information about individual plants with pharmaceutical and botanical findings. Typical research available in an herbal monograph includes: the plant botanical and common names, characteristics to identify it, historical use, action of the herb, plant parts used, adverse reactions, precautions and dosage recommendations. Findings are based on clinic studies comparing existing evidence with a manufacturer's claims. References are included. Some online herbal monographs are subscription based, but others are free.

Herbal Monograph Databases

Memorial Sloan Kettering Cancer Center: About Herbs, Botanicals and Other Products

https://www.mskcc.org/cancer-care/diagnosis-treatment/symptom-management/integrative-medicine/herbs

National Center for Complementary and Integrative Health: Herbs at a Glance

https://nccih.nih.gov/health/herbsataglance.htm

Pharmacist's Letter/Natural Medicines Comprehensive Database

Jellin, Jeff M., Forrest Batz, and Kathy Hichens. Stockton, Calif.: Therapeutic Research Facility, 1999. Print.

*Also available by subscription online at www.naturaldatabase.com

U.S. National Library of Medicine: MedlinePlus Herbs and Supplements

https://medlineplus.gov/druginfo/herb_All.html

When Not to Use Herbal Remedies

For small children, the elderly and pregnant or nursing mothers, herbs are safe in culinary amounts but not in high medicinal doses. Children should only take herbal remedies if they have been proven safe. Pregnant or nursing mothers should avoid herbal remedies completely. Evidence shows that some herbs produce adverse effects anywhere from fetal malformations to abortions. Little is known about what may be safe for unborn children or infants. (18:203)

Furthermore, if taking other medications, do not use herbal remedies without first consulting with your doctor. Those with skin allergies or chronic diseases should especially use caution.

In addition, the American Society of Anesthesiologists recommends patients discontinue use of herbal medicines at least two weeks prior to surgery due to risks of drug interaction, including the increased chance of hemorrhaging. (25)

Finally, one adverse reaction to herbs that anyone can experience is **photosensitivity.** The skin's natural protection can be weakened by some herbs, causing it to be more vulnerable to the sun. The result is inflammation like sunburn and an increased risk of skin cancer. **Photodermatitis** could also develop, an abnormal immune system reaction to ultraviolet rays. Symptoms vary from rashes to blisters. Therefore, if planning to be out in the sun for a period of time, do not use herbal products containing plants in the Apiaceal or Umbelliferae family (known as the celery, carrot or parsley family). There are other herbs that cause photosensitivity as well. Some common ones are St. John's wort and citrus fruits. (12,19)

If you experience any adverse reactions to herbal remedies, always discontinue use. When in doubt, do not use them. Consult with your doctor first.

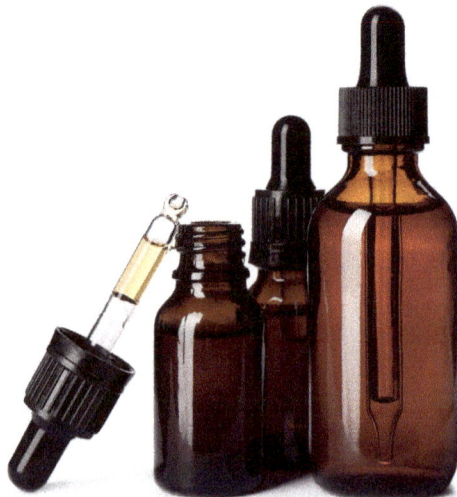

Preparation of Herbal Products

Prior to working with an unfamiliar plant species, it is important to educate yourself. Some plant parts may be toxic if ingested. Be sure to use the correct parts of the plant in question. (See *Recommended Resources*.)

When preparing herbal products, the best way to discourage bacterial contamination is by using clean hands, a clean workspace and clean tools.

Lastly, keep record of an herbal product's shelf life. According to information derived from The Herbal Academy, the shelf-life of herbal products depends on the solvent used and how long it takes for microbial growth. Other factors can also affect shelf life, from preparation to storage. In the case of oil, expiration depends on rancidity, or oxidation, more than bacteria. (27)

For some general rules of thumb, bacteria grow quickly in water, so any product using water will not stay acceptable for more than a few days. Creams and lotions may last 1-2 weeks if refrigerated. For other products, six months is a safe expiration date. Products may be good for longer if made with dried herbs rather than fresh. Alcohol also slows decomposition and bacterial growth. Therefore, products using alcohol may last up to two years. Nevertheless, when in doubt, throw it out.

Remember Who You Are

Herbs are not miracle drugs. You can live without them! You have a loving Savior who, by His wounds, offers you healing. He wants to impart health and hope into your life. True hope will never be found in a plant. Jesus is our hope. It is okay to consult with Him about your health concerns.

I pray that you will keep your shield of faith raised high and always extinguish the flaming arrows of deception from the evil one. You are already free from dependency on conventional medicine and alternative medicine. Your life is not in a doctor's hands. You are a child of the Most High God, and your life is in *His* hands!

Avoid New Age Language and Those Who Speak It

Beware of the New Age speech hidden in most information about herbalism. Marketing for herbs, essential oils and occult Bach flower remedies can include phrases such as: "bring balance to your body;" "enhance intuition;" "repair your aura;" "help embrace your spiritual gifts;" "balance your chakras;" "give energetic protection;" "lift your negative thinking;" and "connect to God."

The Lord wants His children to be set apart. Do not use products that may be derived from questionable sources. Separate yourself from those who speak in ways that propagate lies. Instead, be surrounded by people who hold you accountable and can recognize if you have accidentally entered spiritually dangerous territory.

Test the Spirits

If any of you lacks wisdom, you should ask God, who gives generously to all without finding fault, and it will be given to you. Jas 1:5

Finally, remember to test the spirits. (1 John 4:1) Always pray and seek the leading of the Holy Spirit, letting God's Word light your path.

In the field of herbal medicine, it is essential for a Christian to test all new techniques, products and plants against the truth of God's Word, and credible scientific sources when applicable. Do not let even another Christian redefine Jesus or what His Word says.

For instance, if you are told an herb can lift negative thinking and help connect you to God, ask yourself, "Which God? Which Jesus?" Perhaps others have unknowingly come to accept "another Jesus," "another Spirit," maybe even "another gospel," as we are repeatedly warned against by the Apostle Paul (2 Cor. 11:14; Gal. 1:8).

Many deceived Christians in the field of alternative medicine claim to now have peace about their practices, but peace was not their initial reaction. Never ignore an initial sense of warning from the Holy Spirit. It may be that *the Lord your God is testing you, to know whether you love the Lord your God with all your heart and with all your soul.* (Deut. 13:3)

Learn to discern what comes into your life by way of alternative medicine, no matter how small or seemingly harmless. Even if someone has put the name of Jesus on it.

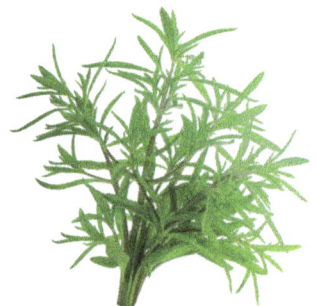

If a prophet, or one who foretells by dreams, appears among you and announces to you a sign or wonder, and if the sign or wonder spoken of takes place, and the prophet says, "Let us follow other gods" (gods you have not known) "and let us worship them," you must not listen to the words of that prophet or dreamer. The LORD your God is testing you to find out whether you love him with all your heart and with all your soul. It is the LORD your God you must follow, and him you must revere. Keep his commands and obey him; serve him and hold fast to him. (Deut. 13:1-4)

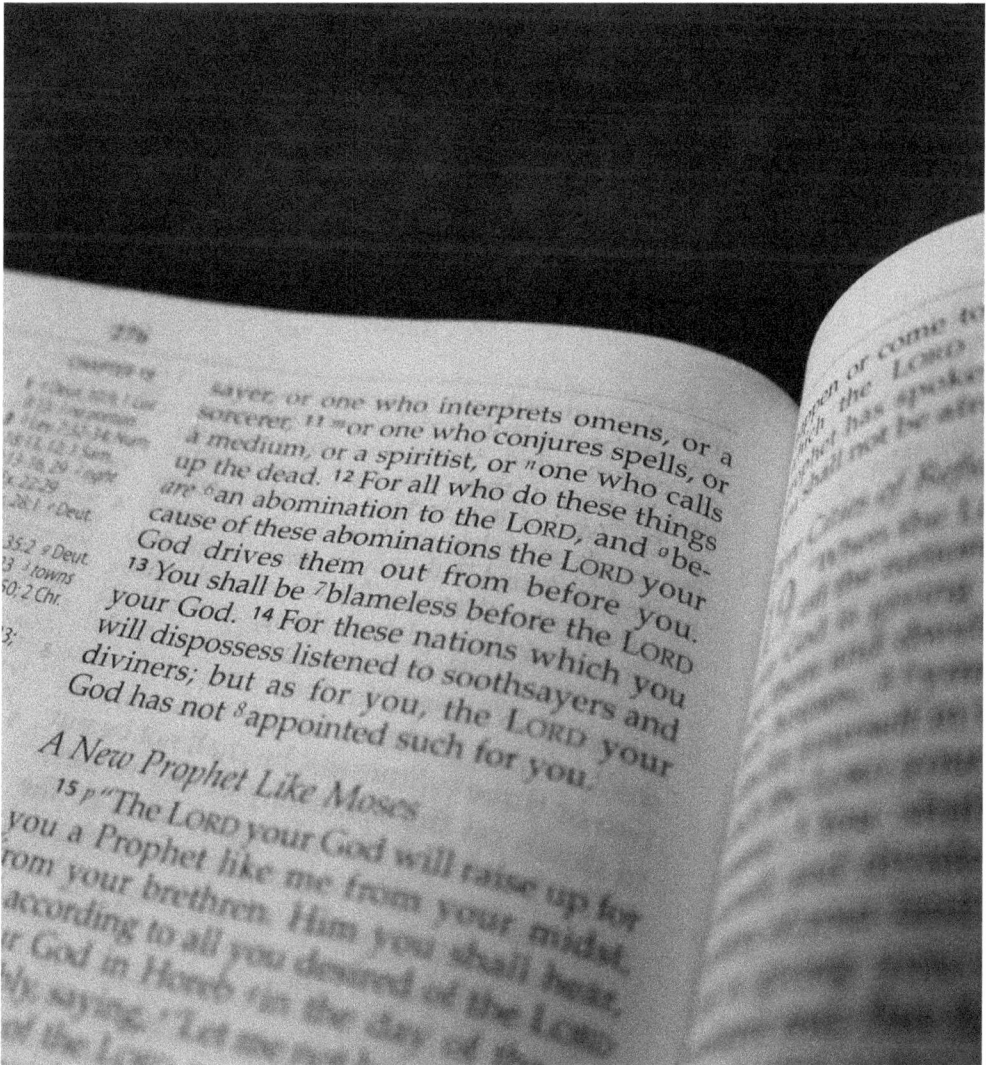

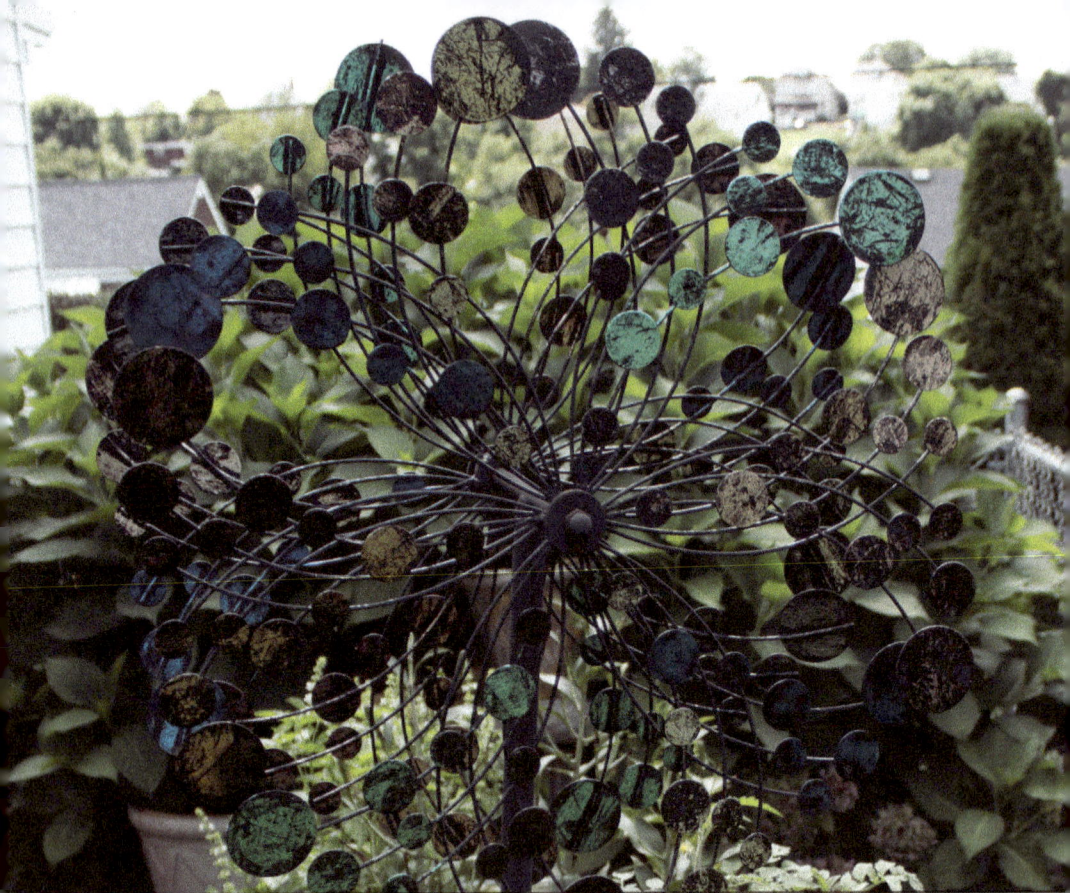

The *Herb Garden*

Now that you are equipped to explore herbs with all wisdom from a godly perspective, let us start at the very beginning.

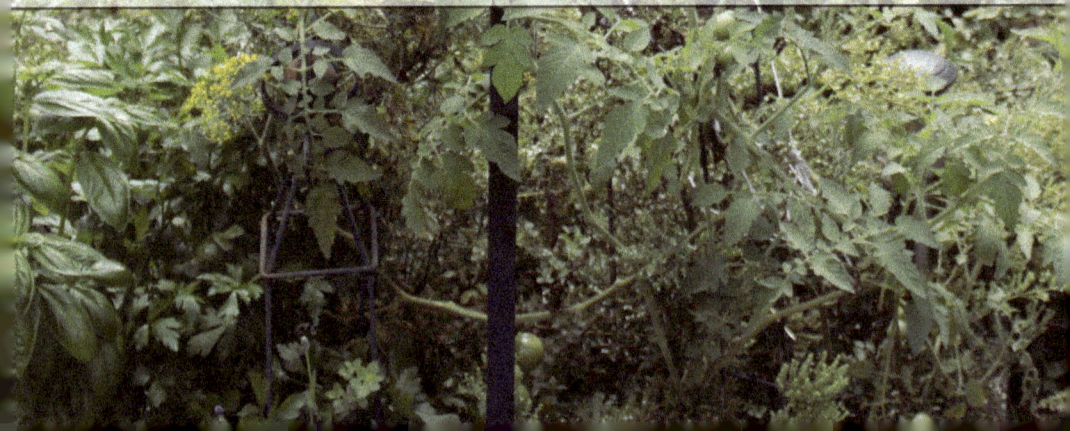

In the beginning God created
the heavens and the earth.
Gen. 1:1

What are Herbs?

Herbs refers to any plants with parts that are used in food, medicine or fragrances. Herbs can be perennials (dying back in winter and returning in spring), biennials (with a life cycle of two years, flowering the second) or annuals (with a life cycle of one year). Some perennial herbs are shrubs, like rosemary, and some are even trees, though these are not considered "botanical herbs" or "herbaceous plants" due to their woody stems. Some herb plants are used to produce culinary "herbs" or both "herbs" and "spices," such as dill weed (herb) and dill seed (spice).

Herbs vs. Spices

The difference between herbs and spices depends on which parts of the plants are being used. Culinary herbs are mostly produced from leaves or flowering parts. Spices are produced from other plant parts, such as seeds, bark, roots or fruits.

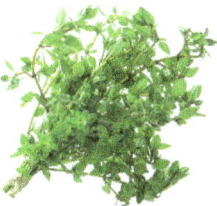

When referring to herbs medicinally, any parts of the plant are called *herbs*, not *spices*, including the leaves, roots, flowers, seeds, fruit peel, resin (sticky substance exuded from trees and some plants) and pericarp (fleshy layers of fruit surrounding the seed).

Herb Varieties

As with other plants, there are several varieties of each herb. For instance, main varieties of parsley include curly and flat-leaf. However, there are several varieties of each! "Forest Green" or "Extra Curled Dwarf" are curly varieties. Flat-leaf varieties include "Titan," "Italian Flat-Leaf" and "Giant of Italy." Each plant has its own unique look and taste, and each may tolerate different growing conditions.

When choosing which herbs to grow, begin with research. Check the *USDA Plant Hardiness Zone Map* (below) to discover if a plant species of interest can thrive in the area where you live.

Average Annual Extreme Minimum Temperature 1976-2005

Temp (F)	Zone	Temp (C)
-60 to -50	1	-51.1 to -45.6
-50 to -40	2	-45.6 to -40
-40 to -30	3	-40 to -34.4
-30 to -20	4	-34.4 to -28.9
-20 to -10	5	-28.9 to -23.3
-10 to 0	6	-23.3 to -17.8
0 to 10	7	-17.8 to -12.2
10 to 20	8	-12.2 to -6.7
20 to 30	9	-6.7 to -1.1
30 to 40	10	-1.1 to 4.4
40 to 50	11	4.4 to 10
50 to 60	12	10 to 15.6
60 to 70	13	15.6 to 21.1

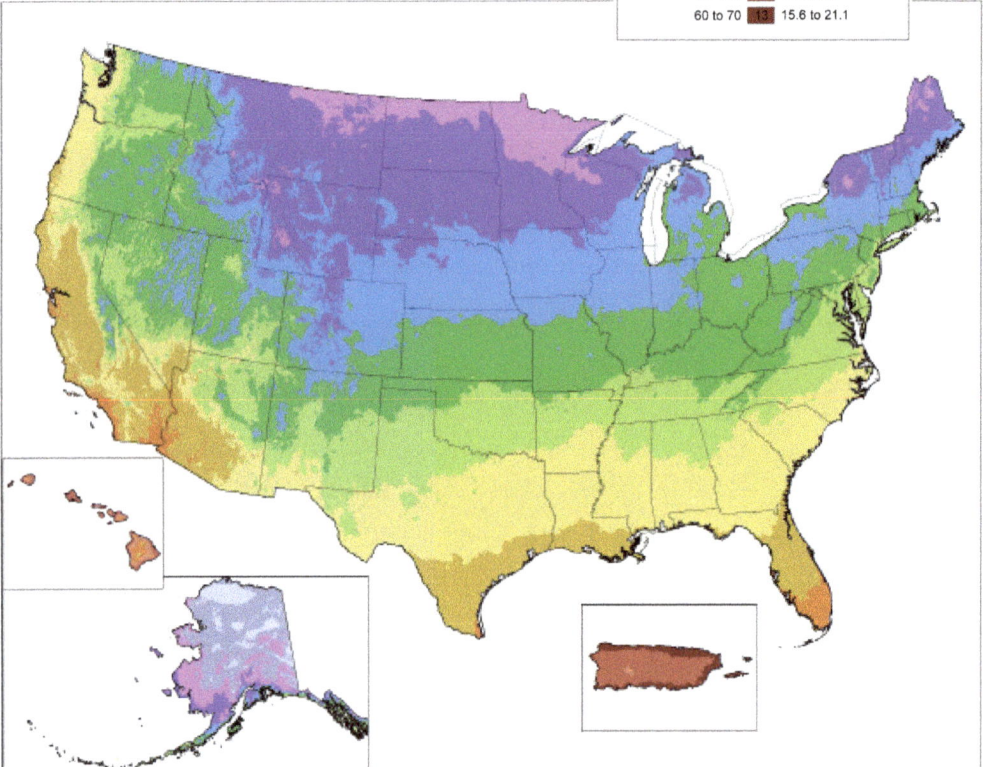

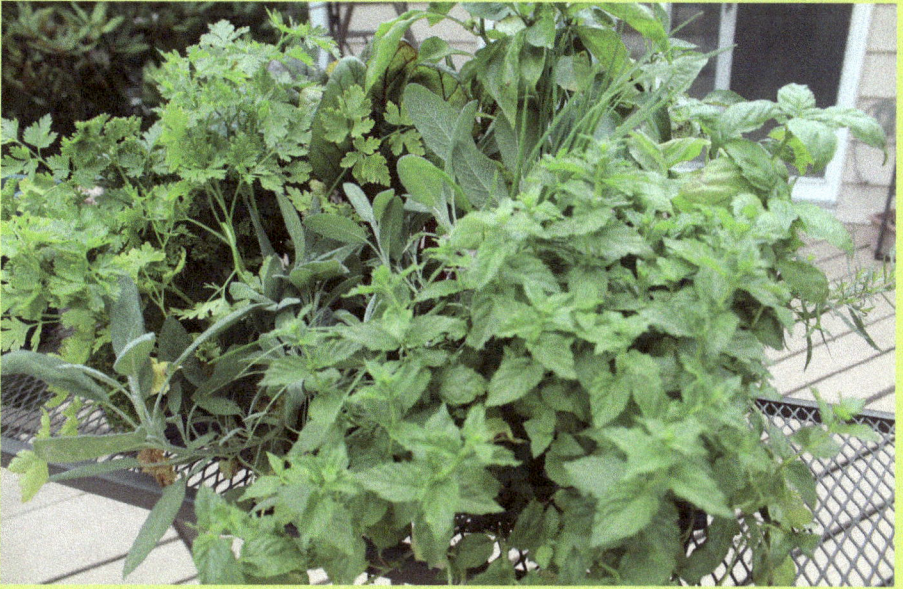

Curly Leaf Parsley

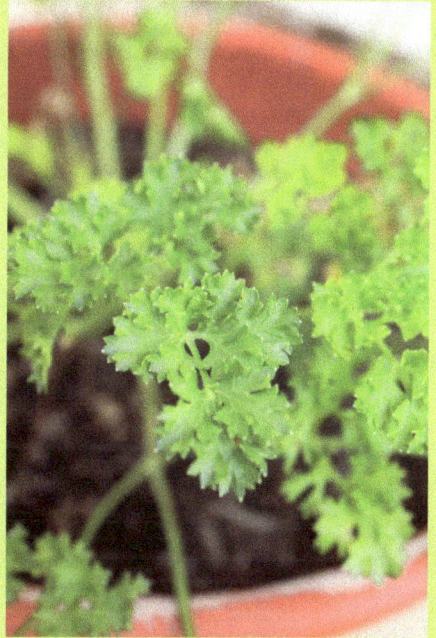

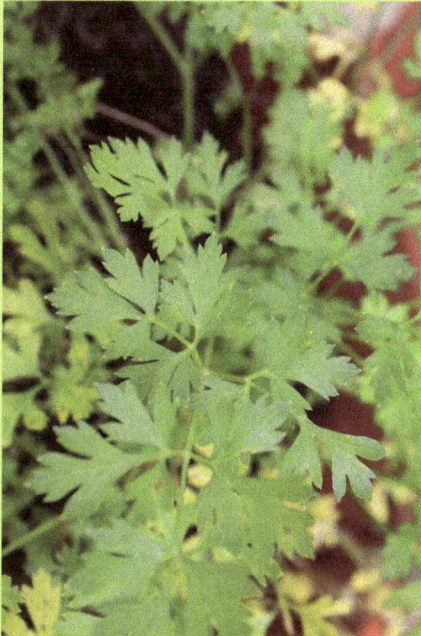

Flat-Leaf Parsley

25

Preparing the Garden

An herb garden will thrive with a little bit of planning. Take note of the areas of your yard or porch that receive the most morning-to-afternoon sunshine. This is likely the best location for an herb garden.

If you decide to do container gardening, use deep containers to prevent roots from crowding. If your containers have no drainage holes, you can drill them yourself. Most herbs require well-drained soil. Be sure to use potting soil rather than gardening soil, which is compact and can choke or drown potted plant roots.

One of the best ways to help garden plants flourish is to prepare the soil in advance of plant-ing. A few weeks ahead, add compost into tired soil to replenish nutrients. The healthier the soil, the fewer the risks of pests and disease. Healthy soil also attracts earthworms which naturally aerate it. The burrows of earthworms allow water and air to penetrate soil. As a result, plants will grow deeper roots.

Notes:

Compost *is decomposed organic matter, such as kitchen vegetable scraps, yard clippings, leaves, wood ashes and newspaper. Composting these items produces a soil conditioner that is rich in nutrients. If you do not purchase commercial compost and other soil enrichers, you can create your own outdoor compost pile. If desired, you may choose to use a bin or compost tumbler. Find a sunny location to increase the temperature of the compost, speeding bacterial decomposition. Compost usually forms in one year. Begin a second compost pile for the following planting season. Maintain a good balance in the pile by adding more "brown" materials than wet "green" ones, and stir every so often. Composting is a great way to recycle.*

Mulch *is also organic matter. It is placed on top of soil to retain moisture or to insulate plants from harsh sun or cold weather. Hay, pine needles, leaves and grass clippings can all be used as mulch. Microorganisms in the soil will eventually turn the under layers into humus, so you may have to replenish.* **Humus** *is decomposed plant material packed with nitrogen and other nutrients that are good for the garden.*

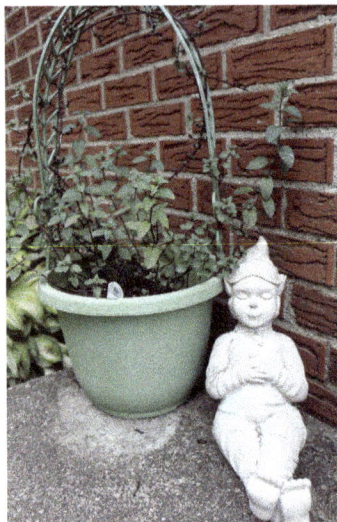

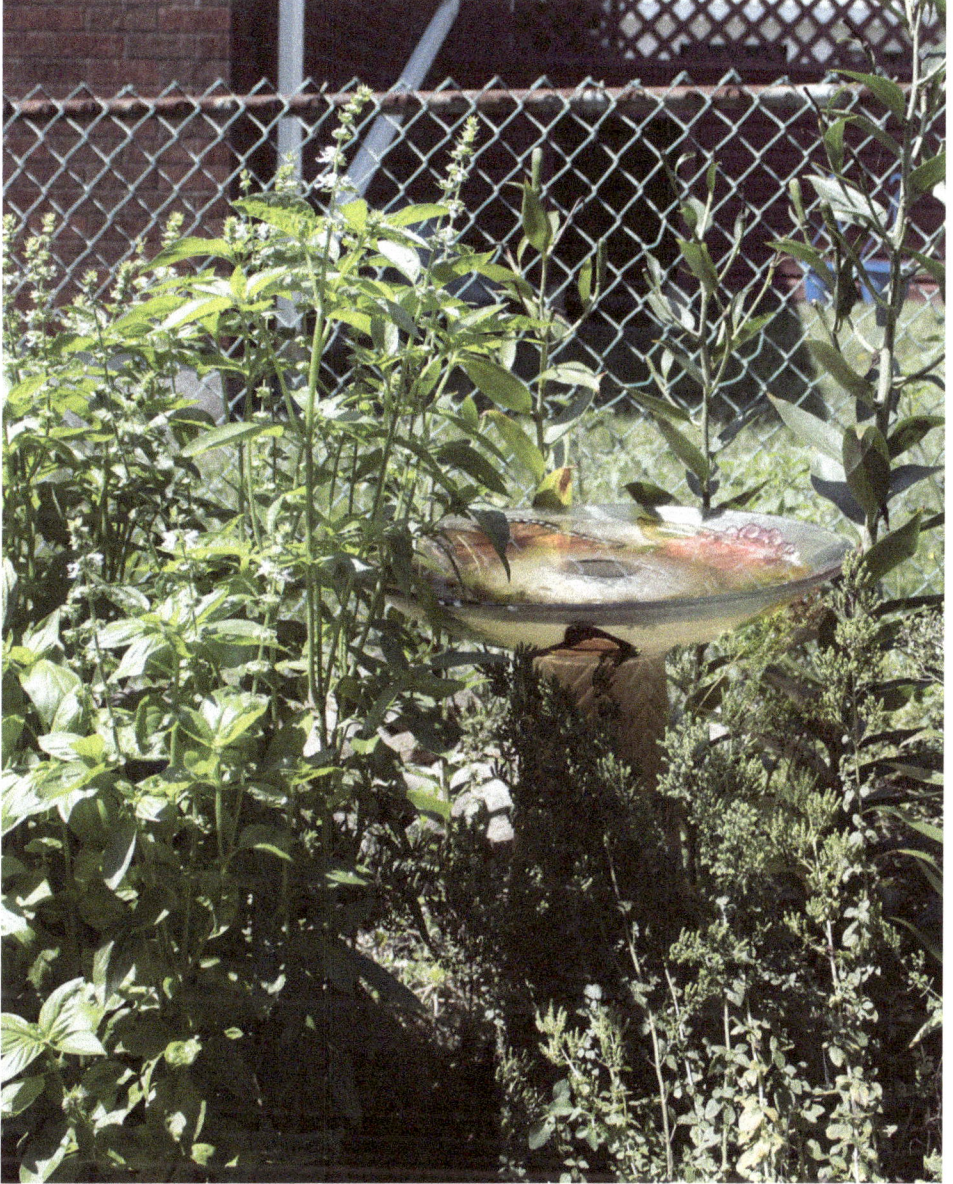

He makes grass grow for the cattle, and plants for people to cultivate –
bringing forth food from the earth. Ps. 104:14

Growing Herbs from Seeds or Cuttings

If you do not purchase plants from a nursery, you can either start from seed or use cuttings from existing plants. Some herbs are more easily started from seed than others, such as basil and parsley. Others may be best started from cuttings or purchased from the nursery, such as rosemary, thyme, sage, mint and tarragon. Researching plant varieties of interest can provide this information.

*Note: Alternatively, plants with trailing stems may develop roots elsewhere on their own, or you can purposely cause it to happen. This is one way to **divide** plants. Lay one long stem of an existing plant down across the soil. Secure it in place if necessary. New roots will grow where the stem touches the ground. Once the new plant has formed, cut the stem to separate it from the mother plant. Dig up the new plant and transplant it elsewhere or give it away.*

Steps for Starting from Seed Indoors

1) In early springtime, fill small containers with light potting soil. Heavy soil makes it difficult for seeds to sprout. Be sure the containers also have good drainage.

Tip: If you plan to keep the plants in containers rather than transplant them into the garden, use larger containers from the start. Some plants, such as parsley, do not transplant well. Research container size recommendations for plants of interest.

2) Sow several seeds in each container and spritz with water.

3) Cover containers with plastic bags or plastic wrap to keep soil moist. Place in a warm area out of direct sunlight.

4) Once seeds have germinated, remove the plastic and relocate the containers into direct sunlight. A south-facing window is best for optimal sun.

Tip: Consider making or purchasing a liquid organic fertilizer that will help seedlings stay strong. After germination, apply a diluted solution weekly.

*Note: If you are planning to transplant seedlings into the garden, you will need to harden off. **Hardening off** means moving plants outdoors for a period of time every day to gradually let them adjust to outdoor conditions.*

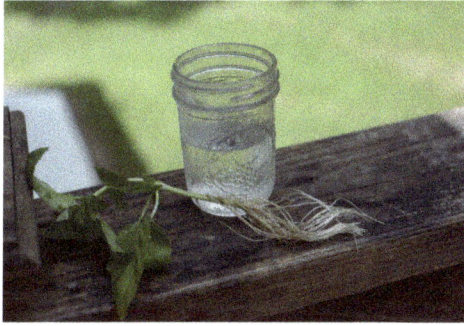

Steps for Starting from Cuttings

The following technique does not work for some annual herbs, such as parsley. It does work for soft-stemmed herbs, such as basil. For woody herbs, such as sage, take cuttings from new plant growth. Older, brown stems will not sprout roots easily. Research the herb in question to know if a cutting can be rooted as described below.

1) Cut a stem about 4-6 inches long at an angle just below a leaf node. A **node** is the location on the stem where leaves grow. It is best to not take cuttings from herbs that are flowering. The plants are now forming flowers instead of focusing on growing roots.

2) Remove bottom leaves that will be covered up, or they will rot.

3) Either a) stand the cutting in a glass of water, or b) plant the stem up to a node in a mass of moistened vermiculite within a potting soil-filled pot.

Note: Vermiculite is a lightweight, spongy, growing medium made of minerals. It does not rot, deteriorate or mold. Vermiculite's sponginess increases water and nutrient retention. Use smaller-sized vermiculite for seed germinate and larger for garden soil aeration. Perlite, on the other hand, is a white mineral made from mined volcanic glass. It also aerates soil. Perlite is the white chunks you see in potting soil that reminds you of Styrofoam.

Tip: If using the water technique, use filtered or spring water. Distilled water lacks trace minerals, and tap water is chlorinated.

4) Place in a warm location with indirect sunlight and good air circulation. If using the water technique, change the water every other day to prevent bacteria.

6) In a few days to a few weeks, roots will form. When the seedling grows, transfer it to a larger container in a sunny location, or plant it in your garden.

Caring for Plants

All in all, herbs are easy to grow. They require less maintenance than a vegetable garden. Once an herb garden is established, simple watering, weeding and pruning will keep plants thriving. At times, you may discover pests or soil issues. Most often, there is an easy fix for these.

Seedling Maintenance

If you have planted from seed, you will most likely need to thin your seedlings. **Thinning** means removing, or snipping, some of the extra seedlings that sprouted so that there will be ample space between growing plants. Follow spacing guidelines on seed packets or information tags. The roots of each plant need to be able to gather enough food and water. So, even though it may feel harsh to thin out baby plants, it is necessary. You do not need an abundance of weak plants, just a few healthy ones.

Most herbs require good drainage. It is best to water seedlings by pouring water into a tray under the container and letting it soak up into the soil. Watering from above becomes safer when herbs are larger.

In addition, herbs love to be pruned. When seedlings begin to develop leaves, pinching encourages plants to continue producing abundantly. **Pinching** refers to the removal of the main stem just above a leaf node. This will cause two new stems to begin growing. This type of pruning encourages branching and will develop stout, bushy plants rather than tall, spindly ones.

Watering

Water plants deeply every few days rather than a surface watering every day. Plants will develop deeper roots if they receive deep waterings. However, if soil dries out quickly, such as with container gardening, more frequent waterings may be necessary. The *finger test* for gardening suggests plunging a finger all the way into the soil. If it comes out dry, a watering is needed. Soil should be moist but not soggy.

The best time to water is in the morning if possible. Moisture will have a chance to soak into the soil rather than evaporate in the heat of the day. Leaves can also dry quickly as the day warms, helping plants avoid fungal diseases. Furthermore, water on leaves during the hottest part of the day may cause the leaves to be scorched by the sun.

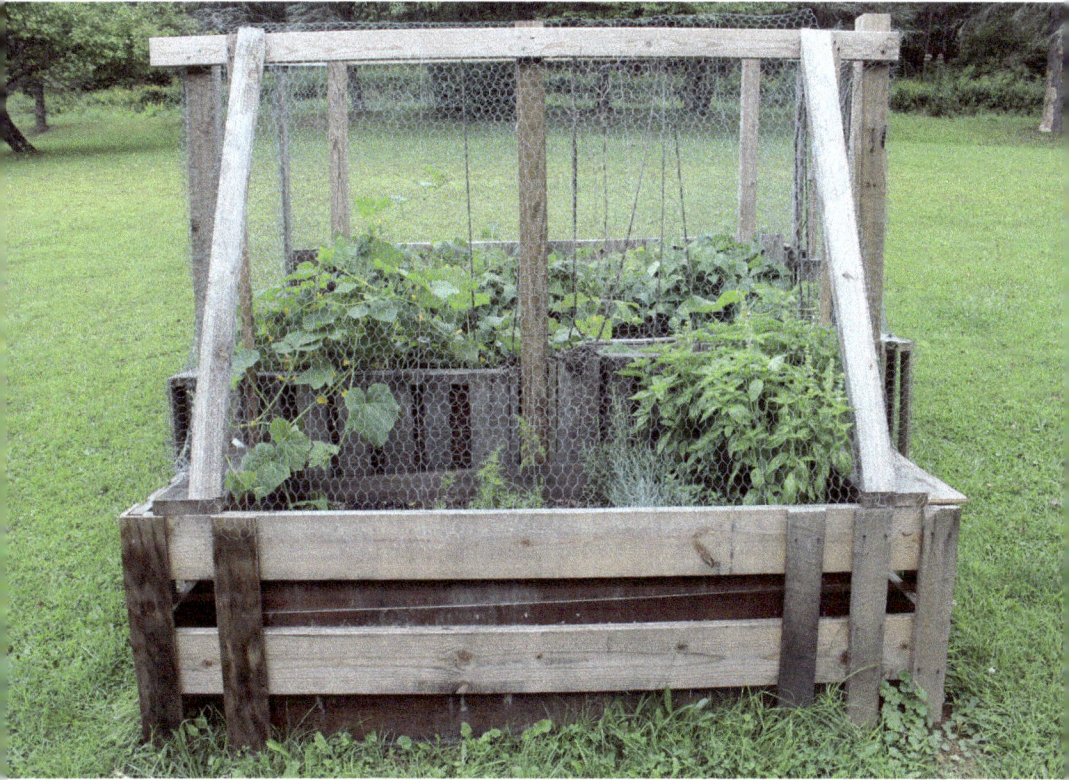

Weeding

Weeding eliminates the competition of plants for food and water. It also helps to prevent pests and diseases.

Weeds will appear when weed seeds have been able to germinate. Once you have initially weeded the garden, avoid turning the soil again, which brings new weed seeds up into the light to sprout. Mulching will also help to block sunlight.

Diseases

Diseases are not often a problem in herb gardens. They are usually localized and can be eliminated by removing infected leaves from the garden area.

If a disease occurs, try to identify it through research. You can then correct the garden conditions that contributed. Lack of air movement, poor watering patterns or unfavorable soil conditions can all lead to disease.

Pests

If you begin to notice buggy pests, it is best to try to identify them. Research will reveal specifically what to do. Even indoor plants can still attract some insects, including aphids, whiteflies and mealy bugs. To remove indoor pests, wash plant leaves with water. Homemade insecticidal soap sprays will also deter insects both indoors and outdoors. Do not use chemical pesticides on culinary herbs that you plan to ingest.

Some insects are called beneficials because they prey on other insects that would harm your garden. If you use a poisonous pesticide, you will also kill the beneficials that control other insects.

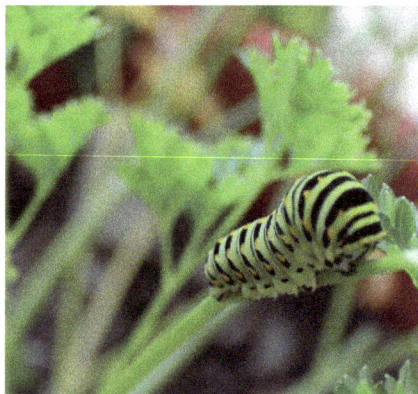

Insecticidal Soap Spray

2 Tablespoons Ivory Liquid Soap
½ teaspoon canola oil
½ gallon of water

Mix ingredients together in a spray bottle. Spray plants top down and bottom up. It is important to spray the hiding places on the undersides of the leaves. It is most beneficial to spray the pests themselves.

Ivory Liquid Soap is pure and has shown to be effective as an insecticide for common garden pests. However, do not use more than a two percent concentration in a soap spray. Test the spray on a few leaves first. If there are adverse effects to the plant, mix a milder solution. The spray works by penetrating the cell membranes of soft-bodied pests, killing them.

See **Recommended Resources** for a book on identifying pests and solving the problem naturally.

Harvesting Herbs

It is good practice to harvest or prune herbs regularly. Snip leaves at leaf nodes. Or, take whole stems rather than individual leaves to encourage bushy, new growth. **Do not take more than one third of a single plant at once.**

Tip: Herb leaves will have better flavor before the plant flowers.

Bolting refers to when a plant begins to grow quickly and flower, and then **go to seed.** When plants enter this phase, they stop producing leaves. This usually happens when the weather is very warm. If bolting begins, it cannot be reversed. Therefore, pruning before flowers form will keep herbs producing longer. Bolting is inevitable, however.

*Tip: For annuals or container gardening, consider planting several of the same herbs a few weeks apart to have fresh leaves for longer. This is called **succession planting.***

If you are unsure how to harvest a specific herb, consult an herbal directory resource, sometimes still called an **herbal.** Online searches are also easy.

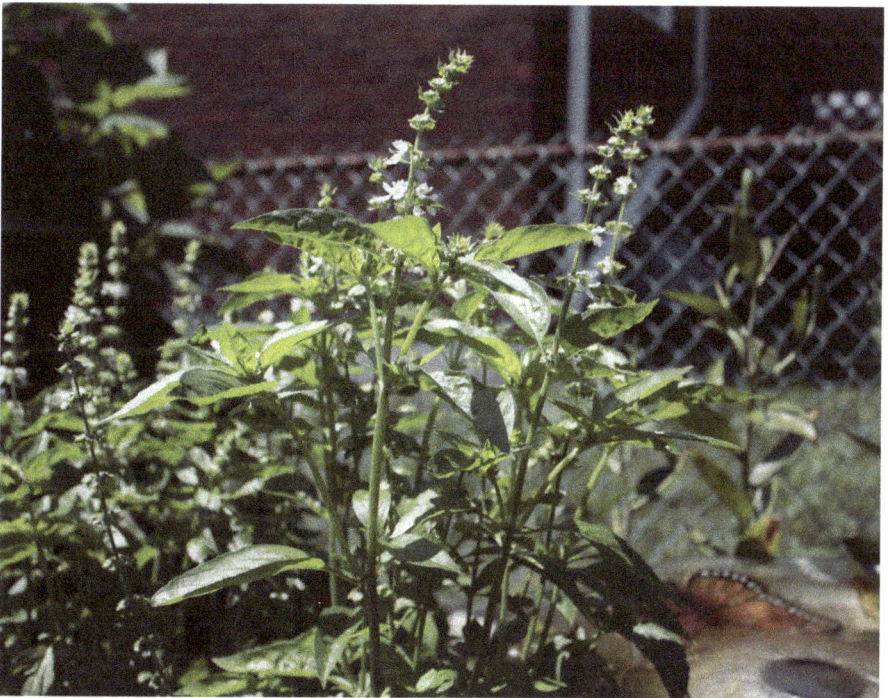

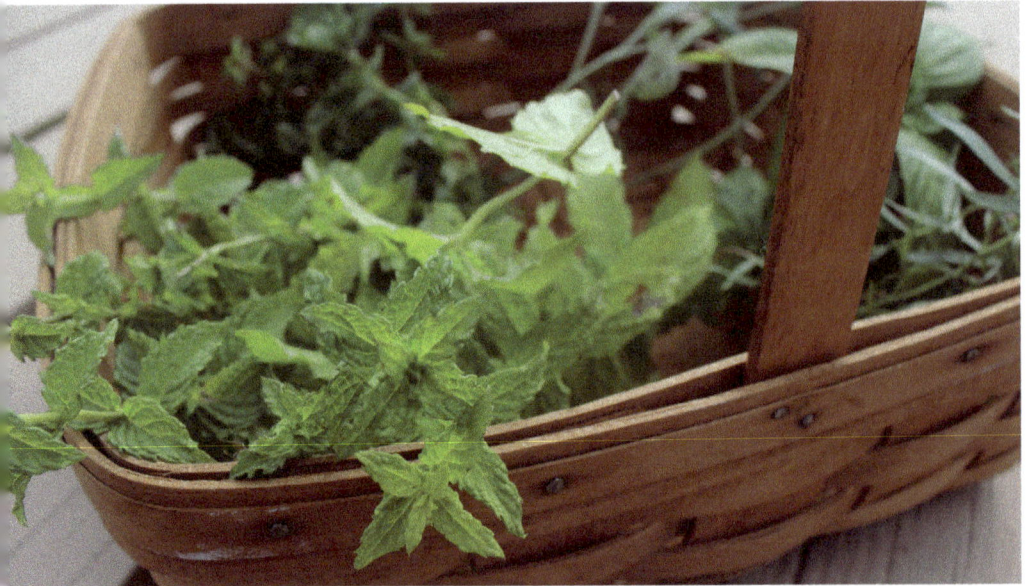

Preservation Methods

To prepare herbs for preservation, harvest in mid-morning after the dew has dried and before newly developed oils have evaporated. Remove old, dead, diseased or wilted leaves from the harvest. Rinse harvest in cool water and let dry. Preserve clean herbs using one or more of the following methods.

Drying

Dried herbs are safe from bacteria, mold and yeast. They will stay potent for 6-12 months. The following are three common herb drying methods.

Note: Herbs are dry when the leaves crumble or the stems break when bent.

Air Drying

Air drying is the time-honored method of herb preservation. It is cost-efficient and works well to preserve the plant's natural oils.

To air dry herbs, tie sprigs into small bundles with food grade butcher's string (or any string). Hang upside down in a dry location with good air circulation.

Sturdy herbs such as parsley, rosemary and thyme are easy to air dry. For best color and flavor, choose indoors rather than outdoors, and keep herbs out of sunlight. Air drying takes about two weeks.

Tender-leaf herbs with high moisture content, such as basil, peppermint and oregano, can mold if they do not dry quickly. Hang these in smaller bundles to encourage the drying process.

Tip: To protect from dust, brown paper bags can be placed over hanging herb bundles and tied closed. A few holes punched in the bags will help increase air flow. If dried leaves or seeds fall away, the bag makes cleanup easier.

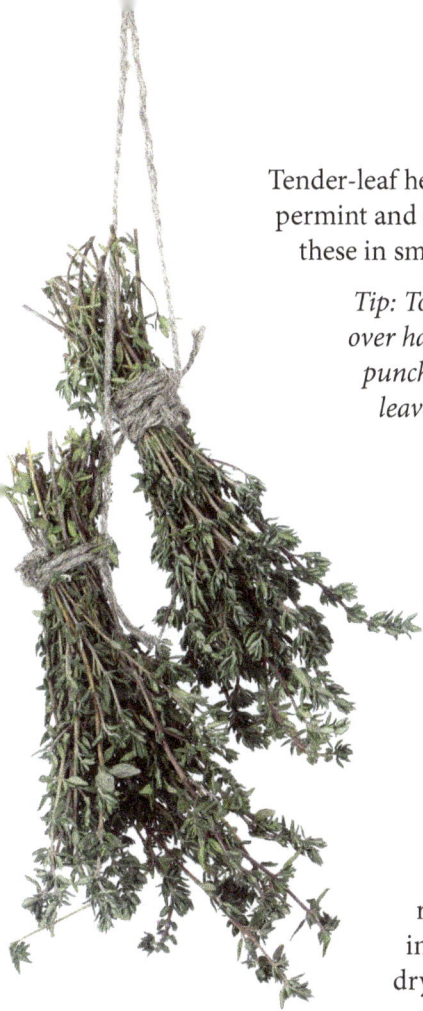

Dehydrating

A home food dehydrator can be used for any herbs. Dehydrators have either stacking trays or removable shelves.

To use this method, remove any long stems from herb sprigs. Spread leaves on shelves or trays in the dehydrator.

Tip: Remove any trays not being used to help increase air circulation.

Dehydrate herbs on the lowest setting. The recommended temperature is 95°F to 115°F, but in conditions of high humidity, use 125°F. Typical drying time is 1-4 hours.

Note: Heat dehydration like this method, or using an oven (below), can affect the quality of dried herbs. When heat rapidly evaporates the water from plants, flavorful oils are also distilled into the air instead of preserved in the plant.

Oven Drying

Since herbs need to be dried at a very low setting, about 100°F, most ovens cannot accommodate. Also, some ovens do not have vents for air circulation. However, if this method is to be used, spread herbs on a baking sheet and bake at 100°F for 1-4 hours.

Ants are creatures of little strength, yet they store up their food
in the summer. Prov. 30:25

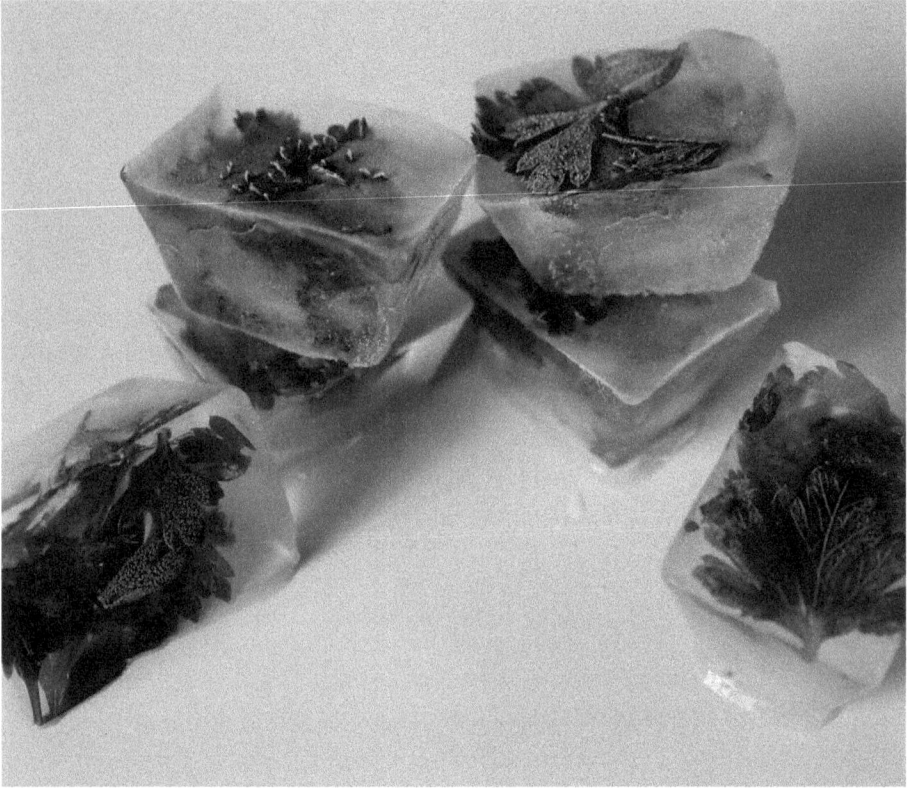

Freezing

Some herbs retain their flavor better if frozen, including basil, chives, cilantro, peppermint and parsley. They can be further improved by blanching first to retain even better color and taste.

Note: Most plant foods are not the same after freezing. They lose their crunchy consistency and are best added to dishes like soups and stews.

Freezing Raw

Hardier herbs, such as rosemary, dill, thyme and sage, can be frozen raw with the leaves still attached to the stems.

Spread the sprigs or leaves in a single layer on a baking sheet. Put the baking sheet into the freezer to flash freeze. Once herbs are frozen, transfer to labeled freezer bags or containers for storage in the freezer.

Ice Cube Method

Chop herbs as desired. Place the plant matter in ice-cube trays, add water and freeze. Later, frozen cubes can be transferred into labeled freezer bags.

Tip: Using hot water will blanch the herbs prior to freezing.

Note: This method makes meal prep easy. Simply add herbal ice cubes to soups, stews and sauces while they are cooking. The ice melts quickly.

Oil-Based Ice Cube Method

Puree the leaves in a food processor with oil to make an oil-based paste. Freeze the paste in ice-cube trays, the same as the previous method.

Blanching is a process that helps vegetables retain their color, flavor and nutrients before preservation. The process calls for submerging food in boiling water, briefly cooking it, and then submerging it in a bowl of ice water to stop the cooking. Blanching halts enzymes that lead to spoilage and slows the loss of vitamins. It also cleanses food from dirt and some bacteria. Most vegetables require blanching before preservation to avoid botulism. Many fruits do not, including tomatoes. Leafy greens such as herbs can be frozen raw, but blanching helps preserve flavor.

Storing Dried Herbs

Store dried herbs in airtight containers in a cool, dark, dry location. Light and warmth cause deterioration. Use dried herbs within six months to one year.

Note: It is best to store dried herbs as whole leaves to preserve aroma and flavor. They can be chopped later.

Tip: To avoid confusion, a good practice is to label containers with the date and botanical name of the herb.

Hezekiah received the envoys and showed them all that was in his storehouses -- the silver, the gold, the spices and the fine olive oils -- his armory and everything found among his treasures. There was nothing in his palace or in all his kingdom that Hezekiah did not show them. 2 Kings 20:13

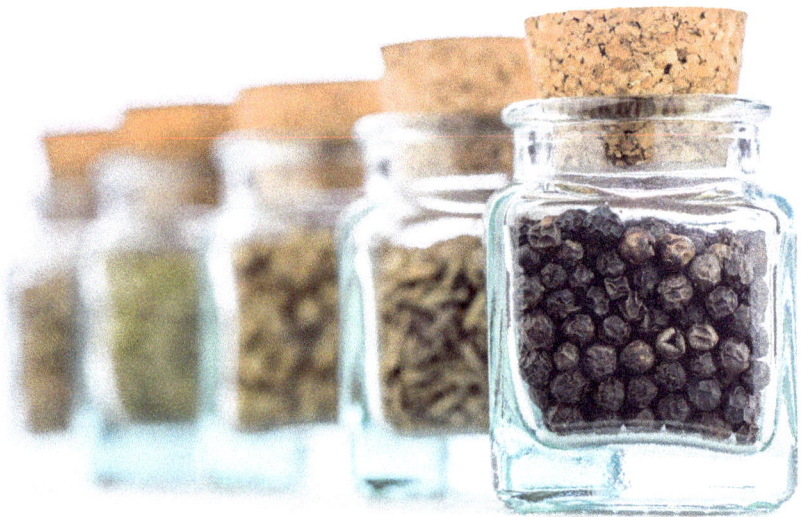

Harvesting Seeds for New Plants

Once a plant reaches the end of its life cycle, it will flower and go to seed. Seeds can be harvested from the flowers of **true-to-seed** plants, dried and saved for the following springtime.

To harvest, remove entire seed heads. If seeds still need to ripen, place seed heads upside down in a paper bag. When seed pods have opened, remove the seeds from the chaff, or dry casing. Clean the seeds by removing any other debris. Do not use water.

Keep seeds in labeled paper envelopes. Seeds can rot inside plastic bags. Store envelopes in a cool, dry location away from sunlight. Refrigeration or freezing is not recommended because seeds that were not fully dried can die.

When in doubt, research the appropriate method for harvesting seeds of the herbs in question.

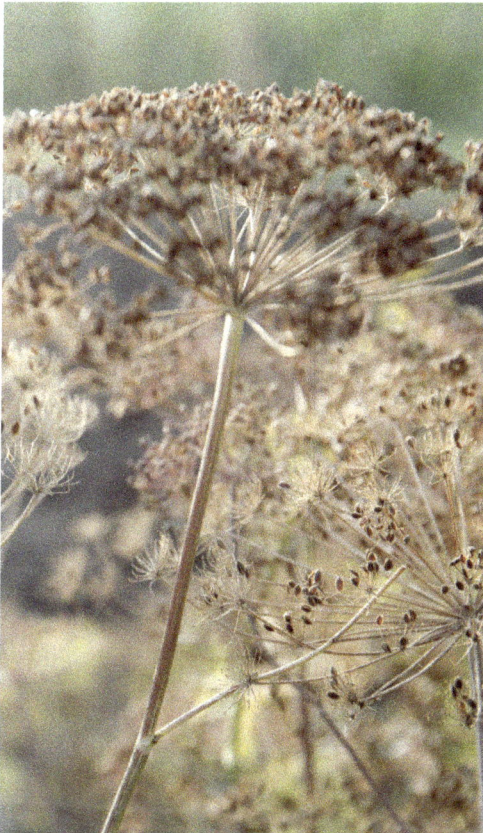

True-to-seed means the seed of the plant will yield the same type of plant. Seeds that are not heirloom are commonly hybrids. Crosses have been made between two different plants to produce a plant with specific features. Seeds from hybrids do not grow true.

The Winter Season

Some outside plants can be brought indoors for the winter though most will not thrive the way they did outside. Place containers in a south-facing window so plants can receive the most sun. Alternatively, you may consider installing grow lights.

For large, sprawling plants, only portions of the plant or cuttings are necessary to bring indoors. Annual herbs can be dug up and brought in whole. It is easier if they have already been growing in containers.

During this season of limited sunshine and nutrition, a monthly spritz of an organic liquid fertilizer is beneficial for indoor plants. Meanwhile, continue pinching herbs regularly.

Note: Insects can come in on your plants and multiply, spreading to other houseplants. Insecticidal soap sprayed on both sides of the leaves will help deter an infestation. (See page 32 for a recipe.)

When the warm weather returns, woody herbs such as bay and thyme can be hardened off and re-planted in the garden. Some herbs, such as basil, cilantro, and parsley, will be too weak to go back outdoors. New plants will need sown.

In preparation for winter, many outdoor perennials can be cut down to the base of the plant. The woody parts of woody herbs tend to not sprout new growth, so do not cut that far back. Woody-stemmed herbs should be pruned anyway to prevent leggy, exposed stems. You can also apply mulch to insulate and protect plant roots from damaging freezes. Mulch also helps prevent garden soil erosion during heavy winds and rains.

If annual plants are left in the garden to die away, remove the debris so it does not become a breeding ground for pests in the spring.

In all, herbs vary widely in how they respond to winter conditions. Research specifically how to best protect the herbs in question.

It was you who set all boundaries of the earth; you made both summer and winter. Ps. 74:17

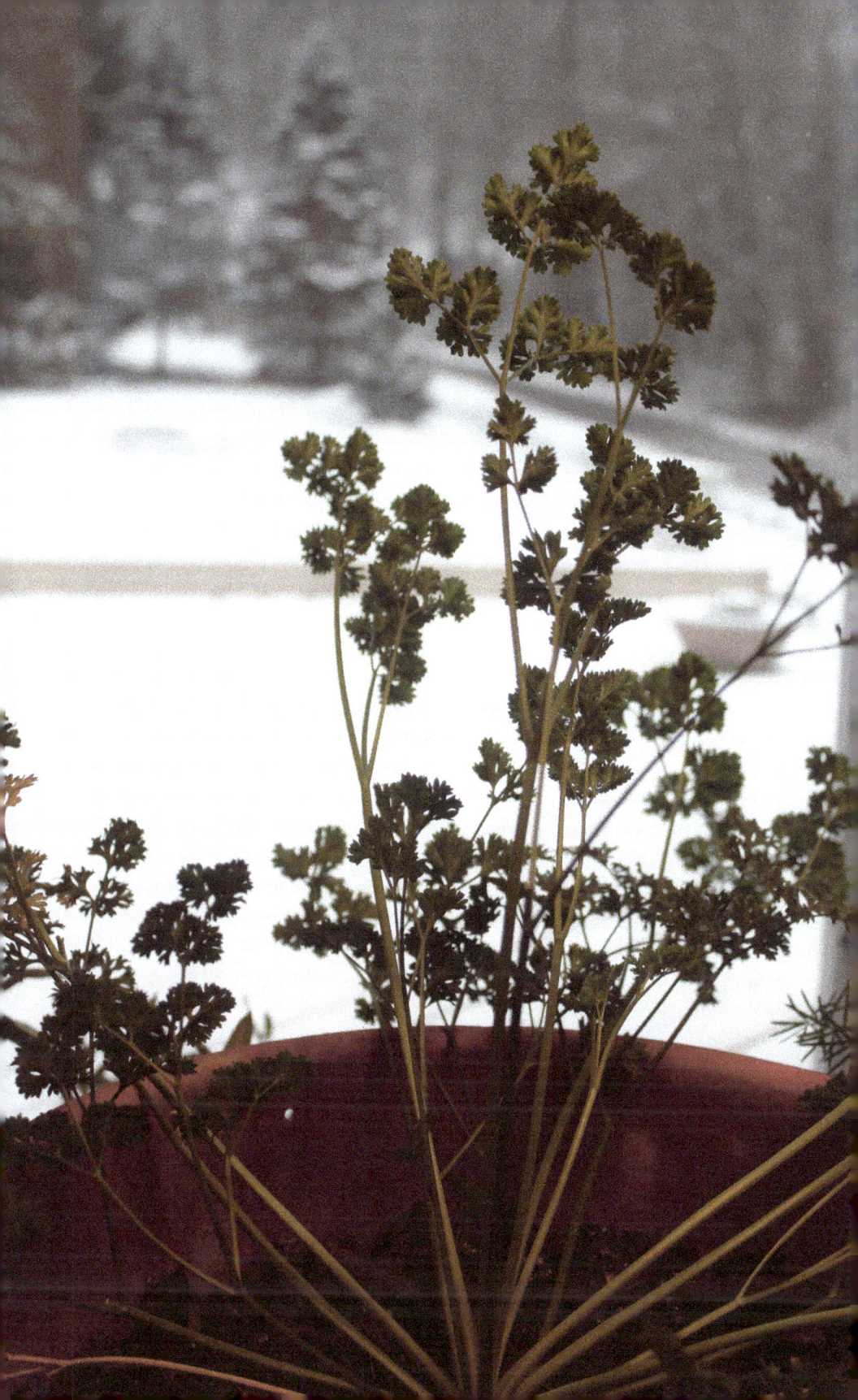

...See how the flowers of the field grow.
They do not labor or spin.
Yet I tell you that not even Solomon in all his
splendor was dressed like one of these.
Matt. 6:28b-29

Wildcrafting

Perhaps you are currently unable to have an herb garden at your home. Wildcrafting refers to harvesting plants from their natural habitat for food or medicine.

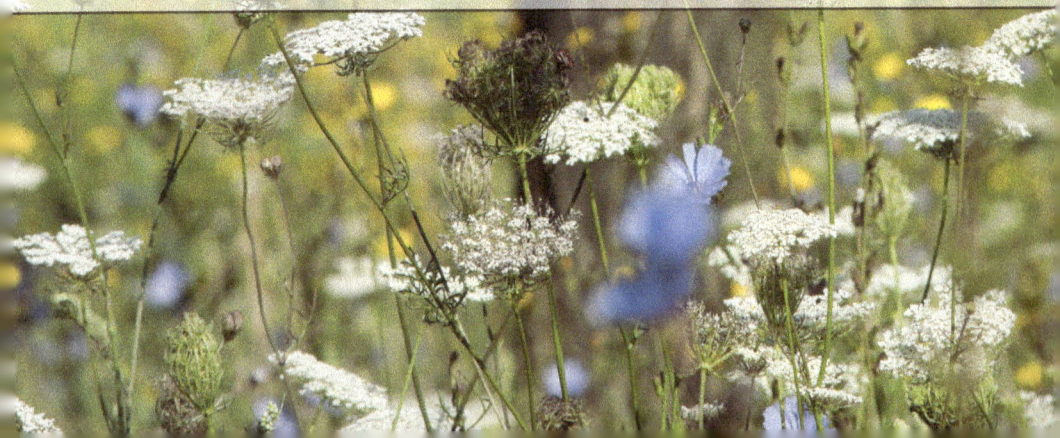

Wildcrafting

Wildcrafting can be an exciting adventure but it takes some time to learn to properly identify plants. A field guide, sometimes still called an **herbal,** helps ensure that you find the right species. (See ***Recommended Resources***)

*Note: Wildcrafting is also called **foraging.***

It is important to become educated in plant identification because some plants have lookalikes. For example, angelica and water hemlock are lookalikes. Angelica is commonly known as wild celery. The entire plant can be used in the kitchen for cooking. Meanwhile, water hemlock is a deadly poisonous plant. According to tradition, it was brewed in a tea to execute Greek philosopher Socrates.

Similar-looking plants are also usually referred to by one common name. Common plant names may differ from one region to the next. To make plant identification easier, Swedish naturalist Carl Linnaeus introduced **Binomial Nomenclature** in the mid-1700s as the naming system for all plants and animals. All plants have been given a Latin botanical name to describe their genus and species. Since Latin was a dead language, Linnaeus would not insult any nation with his choice of language for the system. The **genus** can be compared to a sur name, though it is listed first. The genus groups plants into specific families. The **species** can be compared to an individual's first name. It identifies which specific plant in the family is meant.

If you are interested in a plant's specific properties, you will want to be sure you have found the correct species.

Wildcrafting Notes:

- Some herbs have been harvested to near extinction. If you are only interested in leaves or flowers, harvest just those parts so the plant may live. (3:19)

- Harvesting in national parks is illegal.

- Avoid harvesting plants from the roadside or other polluted areas.

- See ***Recommended Resources*** for a field guide to identify wildflowers.

Using Herbs

How to bring herbs to the table, and everywhere else.

Then God said, "I give you every seed-bearing plant on the face of the whole earth and every tree that has fruit with seed in it. They will be yours for food. Gen. 1:29

Culinary Herbs in the Kitchen

Basil is most often associated with Mediterranean foods and Italian sauces. Parsley is used in soups and salads and sprinkled as a garnish. Cilantro is a staple of both Latin and some Asian cooking. Thyme is used in French cuisine. And on it goes!

Using herbs in the kitchen is easy once you begin. Add herbs to salads, sauces and stocks. Bake them into breads. Mix them into butters. From seasonings to garnishes, let your imagination carry you along. Not only do herbs add flavor, but they are also full of vitamins and minerals.

To use culinary herbs in the kitchen, rinse fresh leaves with water to remove dirt. Let dry. Remove stems. Chop leaves if needed.

Tip: A quick and easy way to remove leaves from some sprigs is to turn the sprig upside down, pinch two fingers together on the "top" of the stem and run them all the way down. The leaves will pop off in one swoop. This method works with some small, leafy sprigs.

There are so many herbs that often no single source gives details about them all. It may take a bit of effort to gain understanding about all the herbs you wish to use, but do not be discouraged. If you are unsure how to prepare or use particular herbs, a little research will quickly shed light.

Tip: Kitchen shears come in handy! Quickly and easily snip fresh herb leaves into foods if you do not wish to dirty the knife and cutting board.

Dried Herbs vs. Fresh Herbs

To use dried herbs in recipes that call for fresh ones, use half the amount. Oils in dried herbs are more concentrated.

Common Kitchen Herbs & Spices

Basil
Common in Italian and Greek dishes; pastas, pesto, salads and soups

Chamomile
Flavoring in teas and desserts

Chives
Leaves in salads and soups; flowers as garnishes or salad toppings

Cilantro (the Spanish word) / Coriander (from the French word)
Common in Latin cuisine; or in Asian cuisine, roots are used to make Thai curry pastes

Coriander Seeds (spice; the plant is called coriander once it has gone to seed)
Subtle sweet-and-sour flavor; both sweet and savory dishes

Cinnamon (spice)
Beverages, desserts, fruited beef and lamb stew

Cloves (spice)
Bitter, strong taste; often accompanies cinnamon

Cumin (spice)
Nutty, spicy taste; a primary ingredient in curry and chili powders

Dill (yields both herbs & spices)
A pleasant anise-like flavor; seafood, soups, salads and sauces; dill pickling

Fennel (yields both herbs and spices)
Slightly sweet, slightly spicy anise flavor; the plant is sometimes used as a vegetable; used in Italian sausages and sweet pickles

Garlic
Pungent, spicy flavor that mellows with cooking

Ginger (spice)
Light spice, mellow sweetness; flavors desserts, fruit salads and drinks

Jasmine (spice)
Sweet flavor; teas, cookies, cupcakes, scones, syrups and dressings

Lavender
Flavoring for meats; teas and baking

Marjoram
Milder flavor than Greek oregano; also in Italian and Mexican dishes

Oregano (spice)
Pastas, pizza toppings, sauces, soups and stews

Parsley
Curly Parsley for garnish; Flat Leaf for flavoring pasta sauces and soups

Peppermint
Mint is a staple in Middle Eastern cuisine; teas and flavoring

Rosemary
Flavoring for pork, lamb and poultry

Sage
Fragrant, earthy aroma; soups, stews and poultry stuffing

Tarragon
Spicy, anise flavor; egg, chicken and fish dishes or béarnaise sauce

Thyme
Add mild tang to fish, pork, poultry and vegetables

Turmeric (spice)
Slightly bitter, cousin of ginger, often in Indian and Caribbean cuisine

Stevia
A substitute for sugar

Flavored Oils

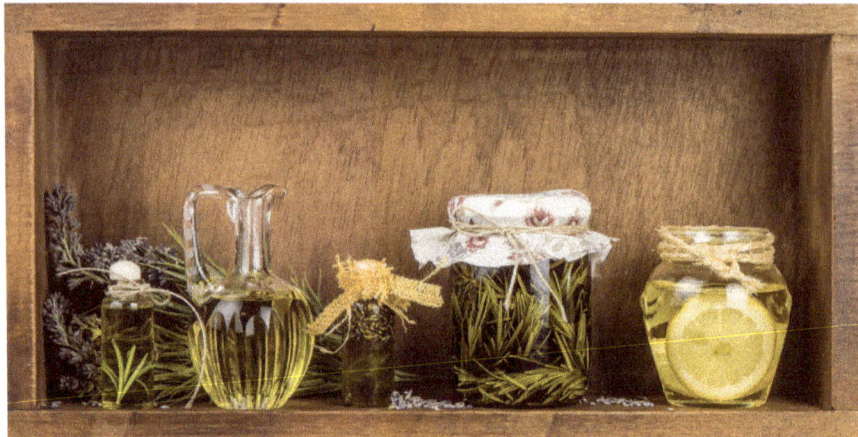

Herbs can be easily infused into pure plant oils for culinary purposes. Make a small batch of herbal oil at a time because it does not last.
(See **What is Botulism?**)

The below direct-heat method for infusing herbs into oil requires heating the ingredients in a double-boiler or heat-resistant glass jar in a pot of water. Otherwise, plant matter can stick to the bottom of the pot and scorch.

Herb-Infused Oil

Start with two tablespoons of finely chopped dried herbs to eight ounces of oil. If using fresh herbs, crush or bruise the leaves first. Simmer ingredients on low heat to taste, at least thirty minutes. Strain out the plant matter using a mesh strainer or cheesecloth. Allow the oil to cool before bottling. Store in the refrigerator for up to two days, and then discard.

Suggested Oils: Olive, Sunflower or Almond

Note: An old-fashioned sun-infusion method also exists, which is not recommended due to botulism risk.

To make olive oil with herbs for dipping, simply mix the herbs into your oil and serve. Or, allow the herbs to infuse into the oil for a few hours beforehand. Discard unused oil after the meal.

What is Botulism?

If you have ever canned produce from the vegetable garden, you are likely familiar with botulism. Most canned food must first be par-cooked or blanched to stop the enzymes that decay the food. Improper preservation allows food to become contaminated, and botulism may result.

Botulism is an illness caused by a nerve toxin from the bacterium *Clostridium botulinum*. It grows when there is limited oxygen, such as in oil. Botulism food poisoning usually requires hospitalization. It paralyzes muscles and can be fatal.

According to the Centers for Disease Control and Prevention, food-borne botulism symptoms show up between 12-36 hours after eating contaminated food. Always refrigerate foods that use herb-infused or garlic-infused oils. Only consume infused oil the same day or shortly after.

Flavored Vinegars & Wines

When herbs are infused into vodka, it is usually for medicinal purposes and called a tincture. (See *Tinctures*) However, wines and vinegars can be infused with herbs for uniquely flavored products. Alcohol and the acid of vinegar both draw out the oils of herbs to produce powerful tastes.

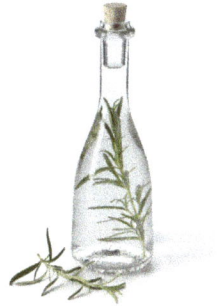

Herbal Vinegar or Wine

Use about ½ cup of dried, chopped or ground herbs to one pint of wine or any type of vinegar. Add all ingredients to a glass jar and seal. If using fresh herbs, do not use so much that they are very compact in the jar. Keep in a warm location for 2-6 weeks, shaking now and then. When the desired taste has been reached, strain with a mesh strainer or cheesecloth. Store out of direct sunlight. Discard after six months.

Suggested Herbal Vinegars: Tarragon or Dill

Suggested Herbs for Wines: Rose petals and vanilla pods to sweet white wine; cinnamon, ginger root, cloves and orange peel to red wine; mint and raspberries to dry white wine.

Note: Vinegar reacts with metals. It may corrode a metal lid or the rim of a canning jar. Plastic lids or corked bottles are recommended for storage.

Infused Beverages

Herbs can be infused into drinking water or any beverage. The longer they are in the water, the stronger it will taste. Steeping tea for over twenty minutes will create a stronger and sometimes more bitter-tasting infusion. To brew a regular herbal tea, pour boiling water over one teaspoon of dried herbs. Double the amount for fresh. Steep for 10-20 minutes or to taste. (For more information, see **Teas.**)

Infused Water

Fill a pitcher with filtered water. Place herb sprigs of choice into the water. Put the pitcher into the refrigerator and let herbs infuse for 2-6 hours, or overnight. Keep refrigerated. Discard after 2-3 days.

Tip: Add fresh fruit to infusions for additional flavor.

Recipe Suggestions:
Basil and Strawberries
Mint and Cucumber
Rosemary and Lemon

Flavored Honeys

Infuse dried herbs into honey to add unique flavors. Rose petals and lavender are popular choices. For easy straining, tie herbs in a cheesecloth sack to infuse. It may take up to two weeks or longer for honey to absorb flavoring.

Herbal Honey

Use 1-2 tablespoons of dried herbs per cup of honey. Strain when the desired taste has been reached. Discard after six months.

Tip: Infused honey can be used as a homemade cough syrup. Thyme or oregano are suggested.

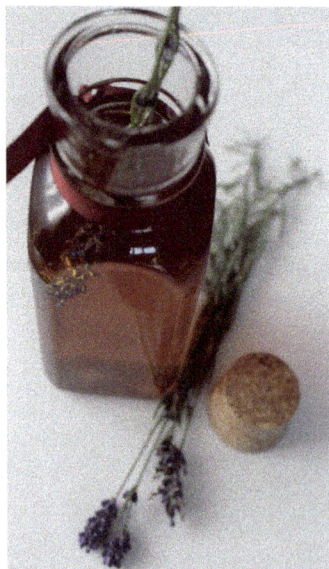

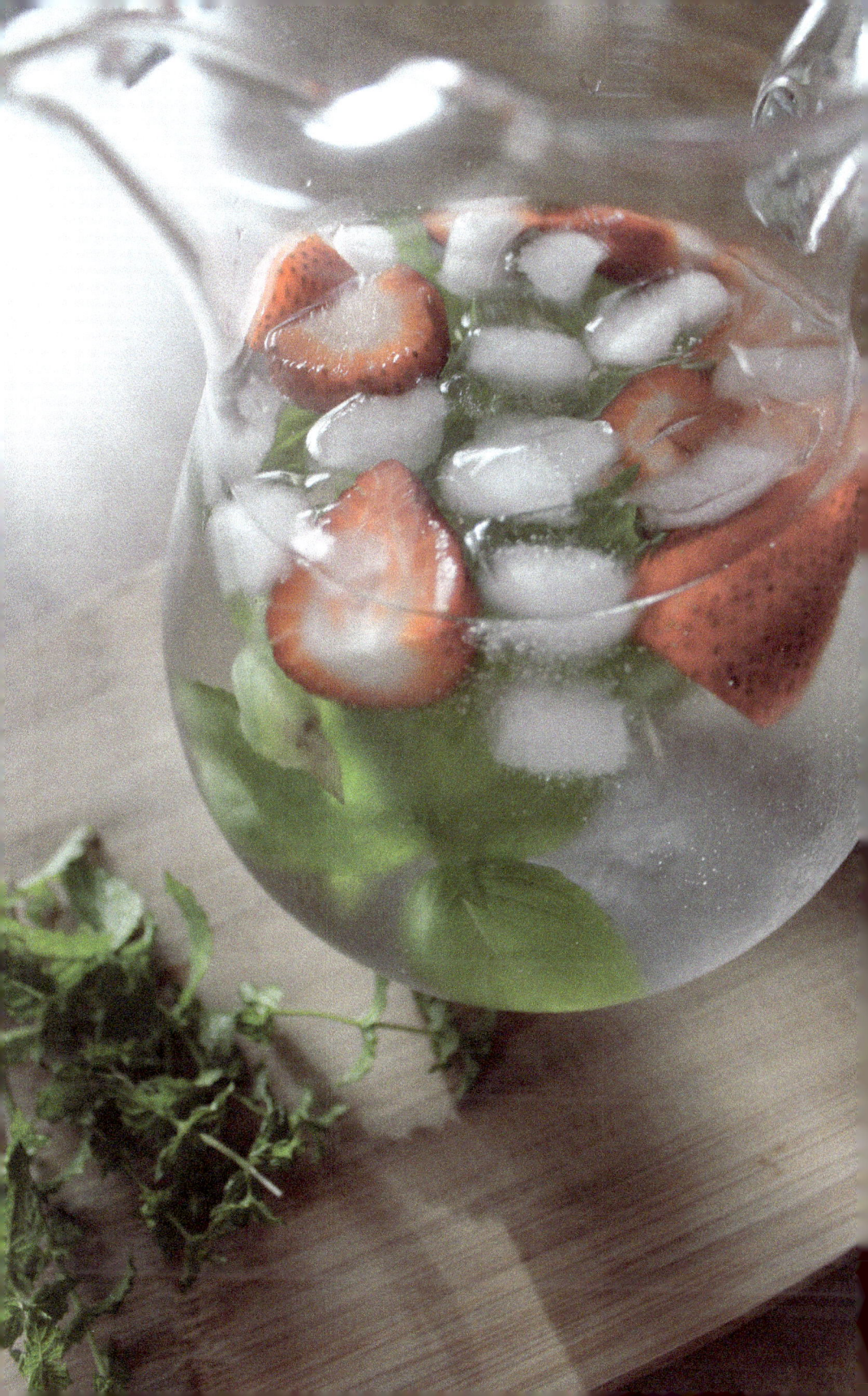

Herbal Jellies

To make herbal jelly, fruit pectin will have to be added to the recipe. Pectin occurs naturally in the cell walls of fruits and vegetables but not in herb leaves. Pectin is a starch that gives structure to the fruits and vegetables. Cooking it at a high temperature with an acid and sugar creates the texture of jams and jellies after the substance has cooled. If you do not make your own pectin, it can be purchased at the grocery store.

To make an herbal jelly, an acid (vinegar or lemon juice) and a sweetener are added to an herbal tea infusion. On the next page is a basic recipe to try.

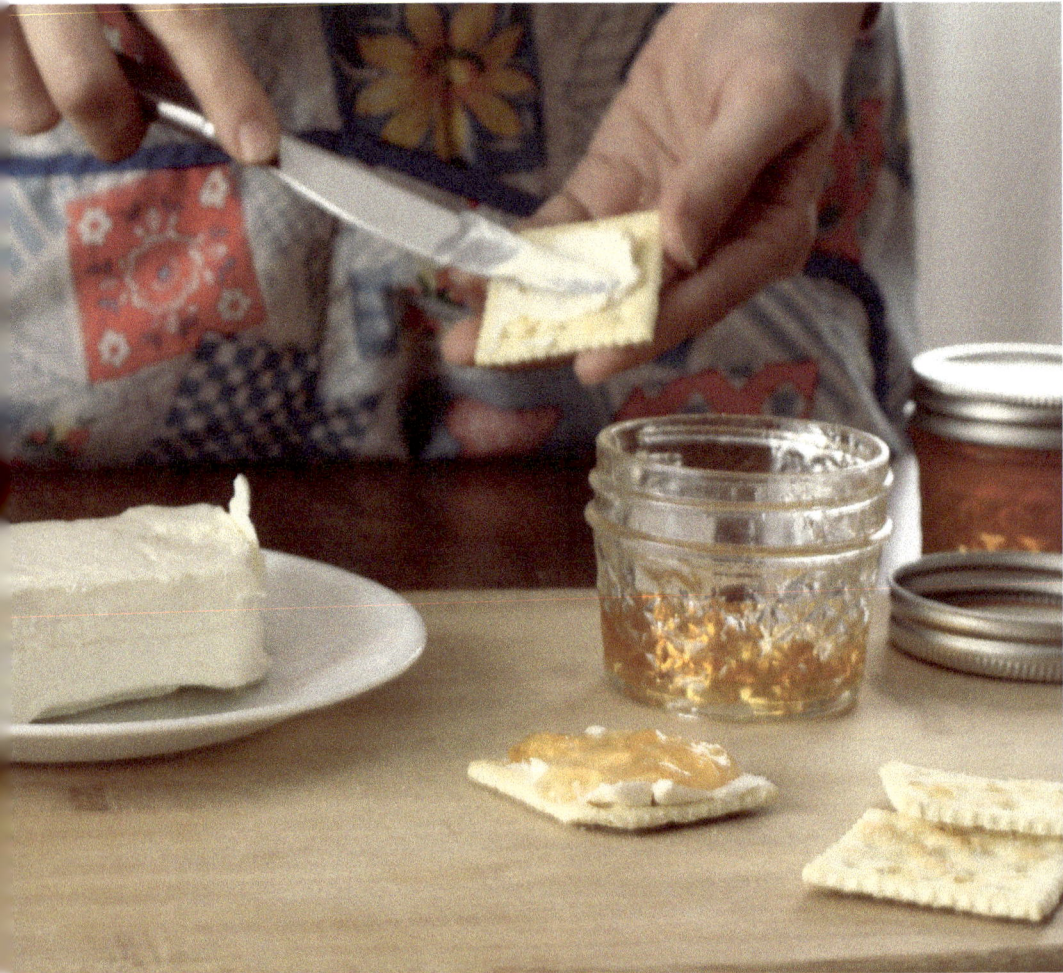

Basic Herbal Jelly

Infusion

2½ cups water (substitute unsweetened juice or wine)
4 Tablespoons dried herbs (or ½ cup fresh herbs)

Pour boiling water over herbs and let steep for 15 minutes. Strain. Add a few drops of food coloring if desired.

Jelly

2 cups Infusion
3 oz. (90mL) liquid fruit pectin
¼ cup of an acid (lemon juice, cider vinegar or white wine vinegar)
4 cups sugar

Add the acid to the infusion. Stir in pectin until dissolved and bring to a boil in a saucepan. Add sugar and return to a boil, stirring. Boil for one minute. Remove from heat. Skim off any foam. Funnel into jelly jars and seal, or refrigerate to discard after 2-3 weeks.

Makes twelve 4-oz. jars.

Suggested Herbs:

Tarragon (sweet)
Sage, Thyme or Rosemary (savory)
Lemon balm
Rose-scented geraniums
Citrus peels

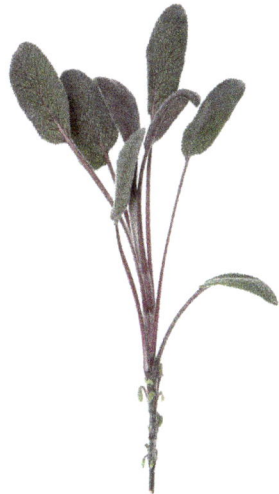

Making the Most of the Backyard

*Every day they continued to meet together in the temple courts. They
broke bread in their homes and ate together with glad and sincere hearts,
praising God and enjoying the favor of all the people. And the Lord added
to their number those who were being saved. Acts 2:46-47*

I don't know about you, but I have always been excited to learn about "the
way things used to be" – and even more excited to put some of those things into
practice again.

A gardener friend of mine once told me how a family treat was created years
ago. When Kathy's kids were young, they only wanted to eat chicken. Her moth-
er-in-law devised a way to make sure the kids were still getting their greens. She
made patties from swiss chard and called them chicken patties.

"They didn't know the difference," Kathy said. "We call them chicken patties
to this day."

Kathy also told me about wildcrafting safe-to-eat mushrooms from the backyard and using parts of plants that I never would have thought to eat, such as
squash blossoms. To use up what is left in the refrigerator complemented with
what is in the yard and garden, Kathy creates a dish she calls "Mixture."

"Do you think you can put these recipes into writing?" I asked.

"I can try!" she promised.

If the following recipes are not inspiration for being creative with your herb
and vegetable gardens and other treasures you find in your backyard, I don't
know what is. According to Kathy, there is "no real recipe." It's just learning to
use what you have. Don't forget to feature your herbs for extra flavor!

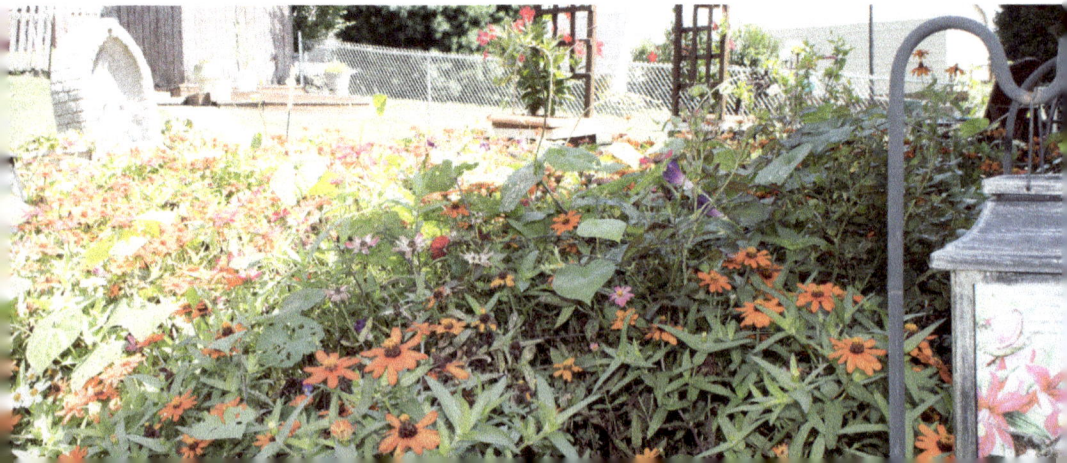

Garden Mixture
from Kathy Bota

Possible Ingredients:
Cubed zucchini
Sliced onions
Green beans
Squash blossoms
Mushrooms
Broccoli
Cauliflower
Sliced potatoes
Sliced carrots
Lots of garlic and basil!
Salt and pepper to taste

Sauté in olive oil in a large skillet on medium heat. (Kathy prefers a seasoned cast iron skillet.)

"You can do all ingredients, or some, or one or two... as much or as little as you like. If you want to add beaten eggs and cheese at the end, it makes a great meal. You can't do it wrong!" - Kathy

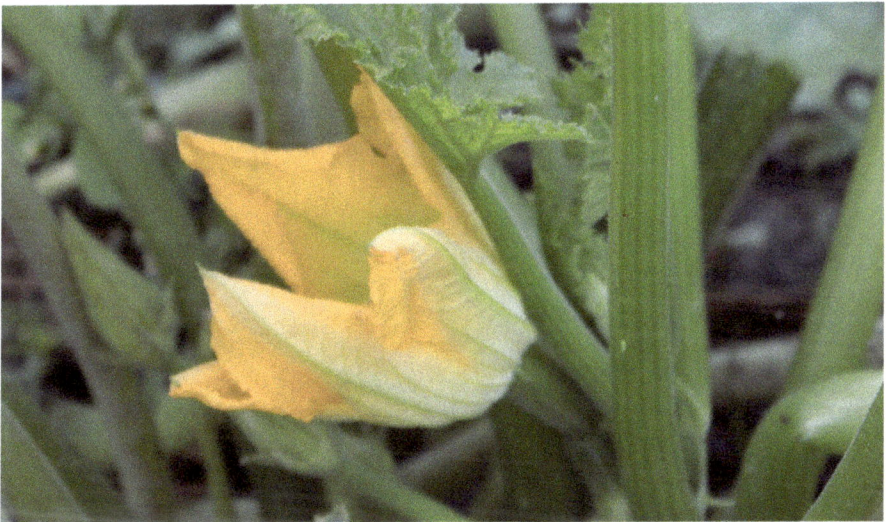

"Chicken Patties"
from Kathy Bota

6 cups chopped Swiss chard
I medium chopped onion
¼ cup flour
¼ cup bread crumbs
¾ cup Romano (or parmesan) cheese grated
4 slightly beaten eggs
I clove minced garlic (or more to taste)
½ teaspoon baking powder
I teaspoon salt
½ teaspoon pepper (or to taste)
Red pepper flakes (optional)
Olive oil for frying

Wash and remove stems from Swiss chard. Chop chard into pieces. Boil for about three minutes. Drain and squeeze dry.

In a large bowl, mix onions, flour, breadcrumbs, cheese, eggs, garlic, baking powder, salt and pepper. Add the chard and blend. Drop by tablespoons into the hot olive oil. Flatten into patties about ½-inch thick. Brown on both sides until golden. Drain on paper towels.

Makes about 20 patties.

"I like to sprinkle with more salt while they're hot. The kids gobbled them up and still do today. Although they torture us about being lied to as children..." – Kathy

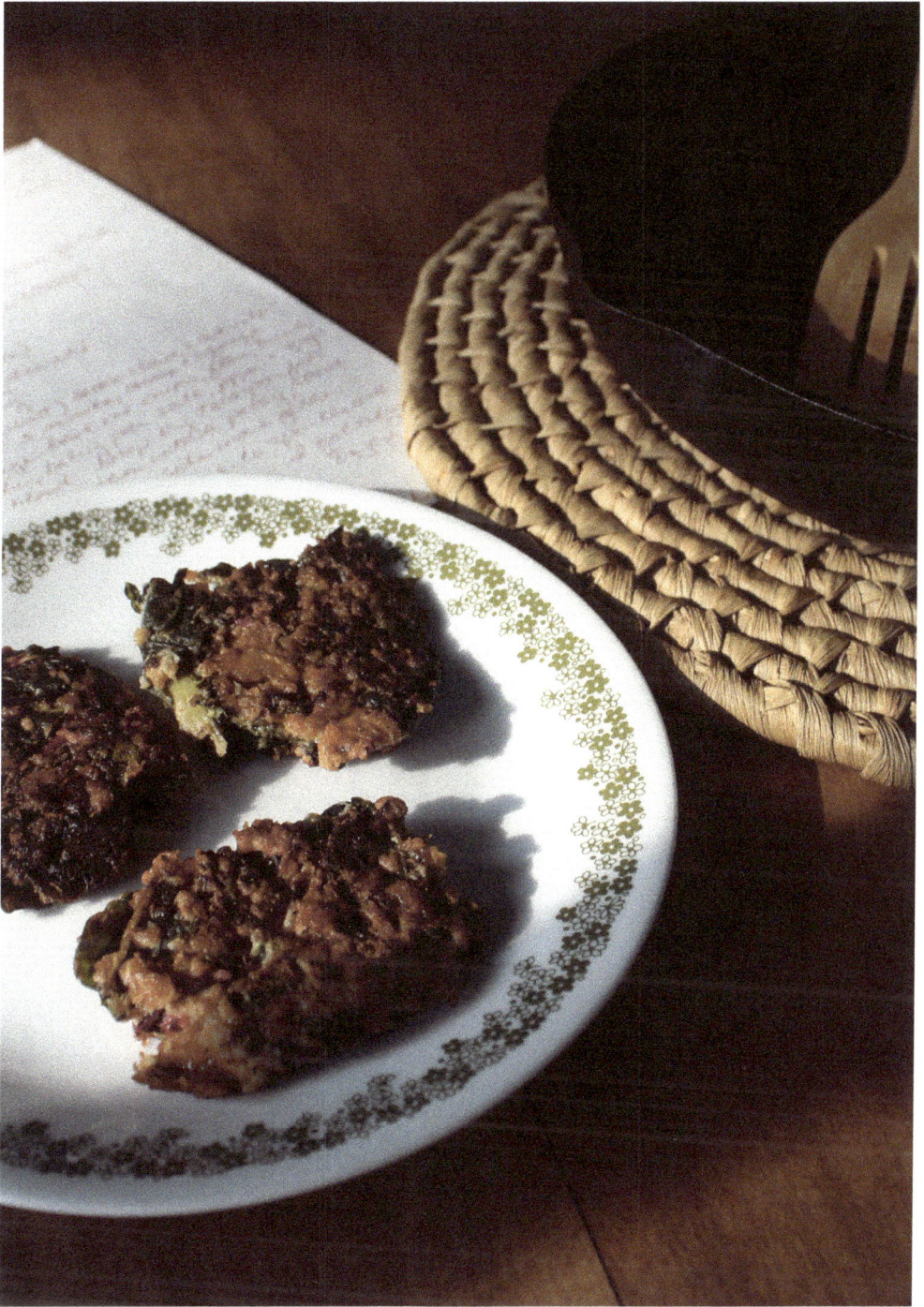

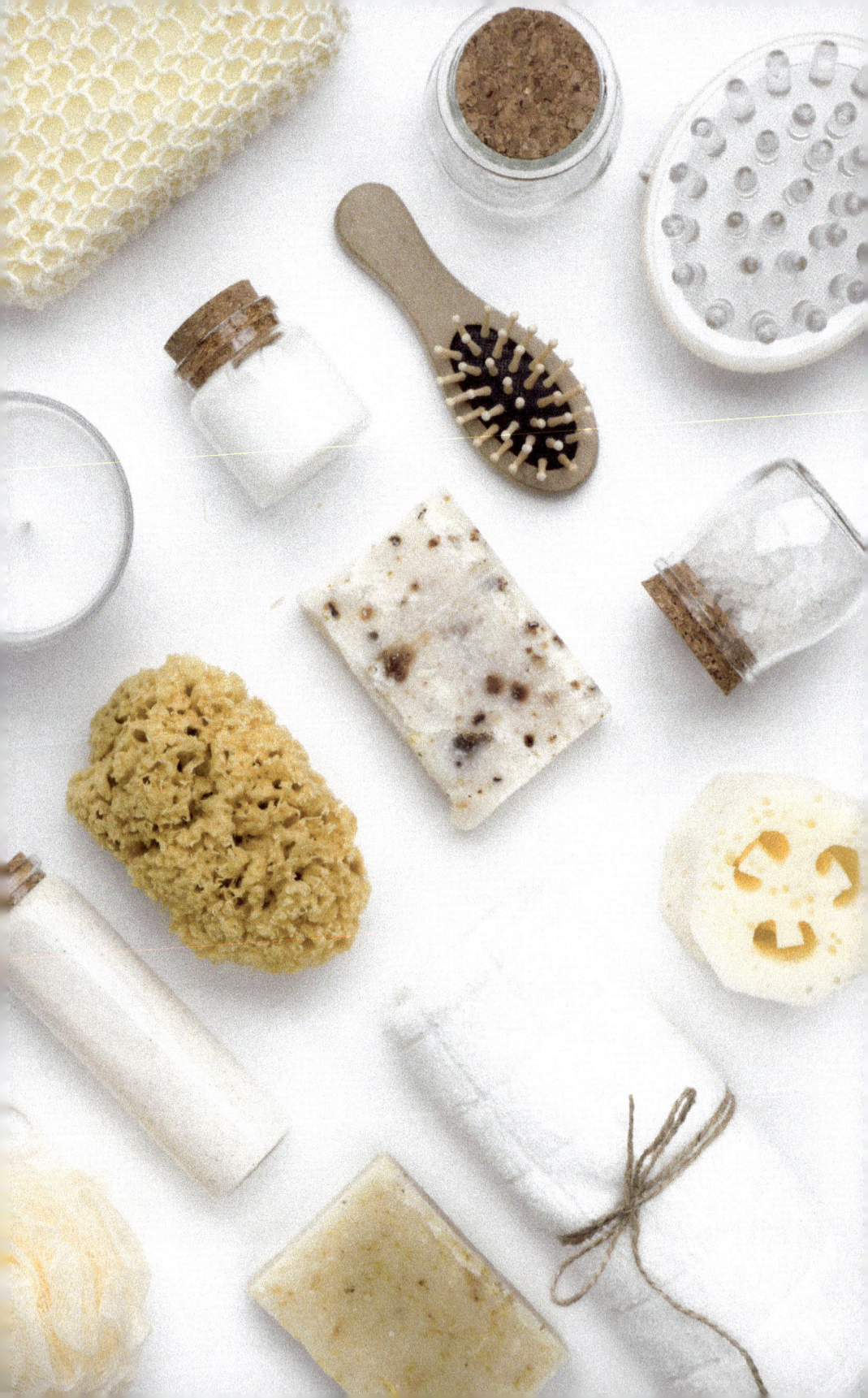

*How beautiful you are and how pleasing, my love,
with your delights!* Song of Sol. 7:6

Bath and Beauty

Your skin, hair and senses can enjoy your herb garden, too. Homemade bath and beauty products are fun to create. They also make great gifts. From bath teas to customized cosmetics, you can be as creative in this department as you are in the kitchen!

Infused Oil

Herbal body care products are surprisingly easy to make. Simple infused oil is the base for many.

How to Infuse Oil

Fill a glass jar with fresh or partially dried plant material, but not so compact that oil cannot easily penetrate it. Add any type of pure plant oil. Be sure to cover the plant material completely with the oil so that mold will not form. Place in a dark location for two weeks, shaking the jar now and then. Strain the herbs from the oil using a mesh sieve or cheesecloth. Store away from light and heat. Discard after six months.

Note: The oil you choose will depend on its use. Olive oil and coconut oil are often recommended for skin care products. One reason is they are least likely to trigger an allergic reaction.

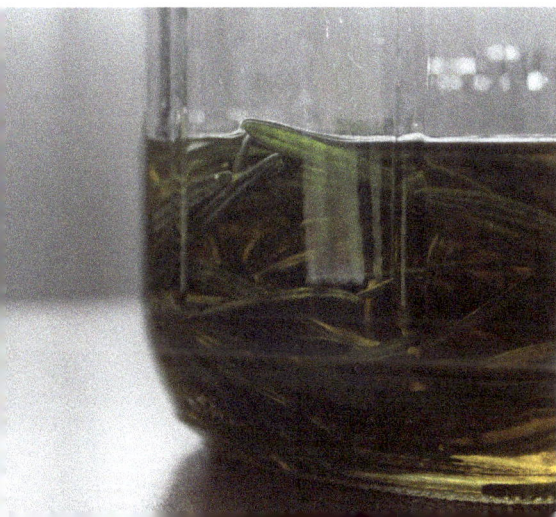

59

Perfume and incense bring joy to the heart... Prov. 27:9a

Perfume

Herbs and spices have been used for aromatic perfumes for centuries. Most commonly, mixtures of plant materials were infused into oil. In other words, perfume was simply an oil infusion! To make your own oil-based perfume, suggested oils are jojoba oil or sweet almond oil. Otherwise, ethanol is used. Therefore, vodka appears in most perfume recipes.

Note: Alcohol infusions last longer than other infusions.

Basic Perfume

Start with eight ounces of vodka in a glass jar. Crush desired dried herbs and spices with a mortar and pestle, and add them to the jar. Seal and store away, shaking now and then, for 2-6 weeks. Strain and pour into a glass bottle with a mister top. Discard after 1-2 years.

Perfume Ingredient Suggestions:
The **top note** of a perfume accounts for the initial scent. It disperses first. Citrus, sweet smelling herbs and light fruits are most commonly used as top notes. The **middle note** or "heart" scent of a perfume can be detected once the top note evaporates. It lasts a little longer. Florals are most common, such as rose geranium, lavender or jasmine. The **base note** of perfume lingers the longest. Base note fragrances are rich, such as cinnamon, vanilla, musk, cedar or pine.

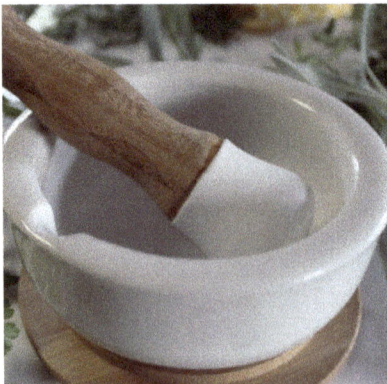

A mortar and pestle are implements that have been used since ancient times to crush and grind ingredients. The mortar is a bowl made of a hard material. The pestle is a blunt object used for the crushing and grinding.

Massage Oils

Infused oils can be used for massage. Herbs are selected based their benefits to the body and skin, such as the anti-inflammatory, pain-relieving qualities of lavender, rosemary, chamomile or peppermint.

Popular carrier oils for massage are fractionated coconut oil, jojoba oil, sunflower oil or almond oil. The term **carrier oil** refers to the base oil being infused. When choosing plant-based carrier oils, be aware of any allergies.

Caution: Some herbs can cause photosensitivity, which is an adverse reaction to the sun. St. John's wort, lavender, rosemary and citrus are all examples. The reaction appears as inflammation to the skin. Do not apply an oil infusion of these herbs to the skin before going out in the sun. (See **When Not to Use Herbal Remedies)*

Oil embrocation of the body was a daily occurrence for the people of ancient Israel. It involved a moistening and rubbing of the skin with oil or lotion. The practice was discontinued only during mourning. (2 Sam. 12:19-20; Dan.10:2-3) The most commonly used oil was olive oil. It soothed and protected the skin. Since embrocation was accompanied by massage, scholars have assumed a therapeutic intent. A bath in a bathhouse was followed by an oil rub. In times of wealth, fragrant oils were used. (20:370-371, 537-538)

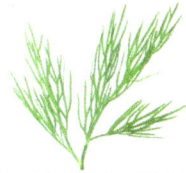

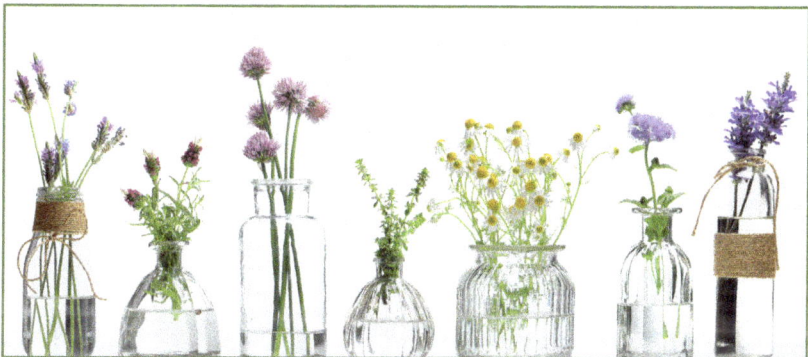

Lotions & Creams

The way to add herbal goodness to your homemade body lotion and cream products is to infuse either the oil or the water of the recipes, or both. The difference between lotions and creams is the thickness of the product. **Lotions** have higher water content whereas **creams** tend to have a thicker consistency. Adjust your recipes as you desire.

For a simple recipe, measure one cup of pure plant oil or infused oil into a small saucepan. Add two tablespoons (1 oz.) of beeswax. Heat the oil and wax on low heat to melt them together. Pour the mixture into a blender. While blending at a low speed, slowly add distilled water (or an herbal tea – see *Teas*) one tablespoon at a time. The mixture will begin to thicken as it blends. Add the water to your preferred consistency. Refrigerate. Discard after 1-2 weeks.

Tips:

• *Have a blender, saucepan and other tools only for making body care products. Residues from products can remain on tools, so you may not want to use them as kitchen tools.*

• *Adjust the oil measurement in recipes depending on skin type. Use less oil for oily skin and more for dry skin.*

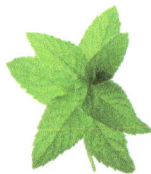

Plants that especially love your skin are: rose (*Rosa centifolia* and *Rosa damascena*), rosehips of the sweet-brier rose (*Rosa rubiginosa*), mint (*Mentha piperita* and *Menntha spicata*), green tea (*Camellia sinensis*), Aloe vera, calendula, chamomile and lavender. Plants with oils that have skin restoring benefits and Vitamin E are argan (*Argania spinosa*), avocado (*Persea gratissima*) and sweet almond (*Prunus amygdalus dulcis*). (6)

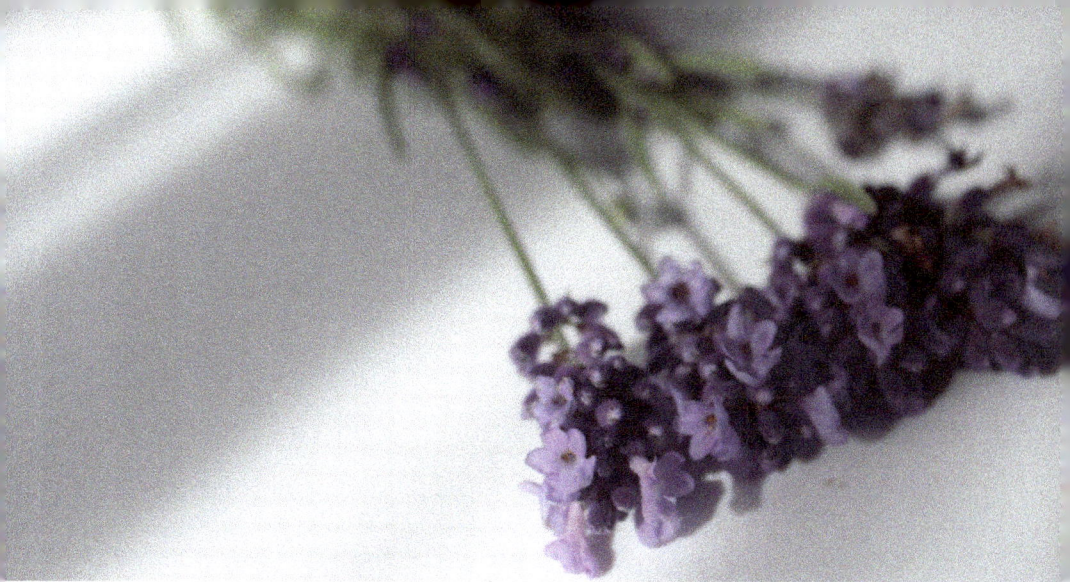

Hair Care

Folklore reveals that many herbs have been used through the centuries to benefit hair from enhancing shine to adding body. For instance, calendula conditions oily hair. Chamomile soothes the scalp. And parsley has been used to prevent dandruff.

However, be sure to do careful research when selecting herbs. Some have been used to lighten or add tints to hair, and you do not want to inadvertently cause an effect you did not expect.

Hair Rinse

An herbal decoction can be used as a hair rinse. (See *Teas*.)

Leave-In Conditioner

To make your own herbal conditioner, add one tablespoon of glycerin or jojoba oil and one tablespoon of *Aloe vera* gel into five tablespoons of warmed herbal decoction. It is not necessary to rinse this product from your hair.

> Women of the ancient world perfumed their hair with fragrant oils. In his work on cosmetics, Greek physician Criton describes twenty-five different types of hair oils. (20:372)

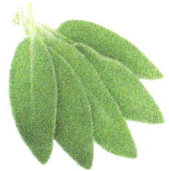

Soaps

Herb infusions can be used in soapmaking in lieu of essential oils. However, the resulting fragrance is more mild. It is also unknown if the benefits of the plant extracts survive the high alkalinity and heat of the soapmaking process. (2:162) Nevertheless, herbs add color, texture and decoration to homemade soaps.

To make soap with herbs, infuse the oil, distilled water or milk ingredients of a soap recipe with your herbs of choice. Refer to the **Infused Oil** recipe to learn about infusing oil, or see **Teas** to learn about infusing water. Infuse milk by adding one part plant material to two parts milk and store in the refrigerator for a few days. Strain the milk and use it, or freeze it using ice cube trays. Infused milk can be kept frozen for up to six months in preparation for the next soap-making day.

Note: Using green herbs in milk infusions may darken the color of the soap. To avoid altering colors, use flowers for milk infusions.

Tip: Dried flowers can also be added to the top of soaps for decoration. Place garnishments on freshly poured soap batter. Press them in slightly to secure.

See **Recommended Resources** for books on how to make natural soaps.

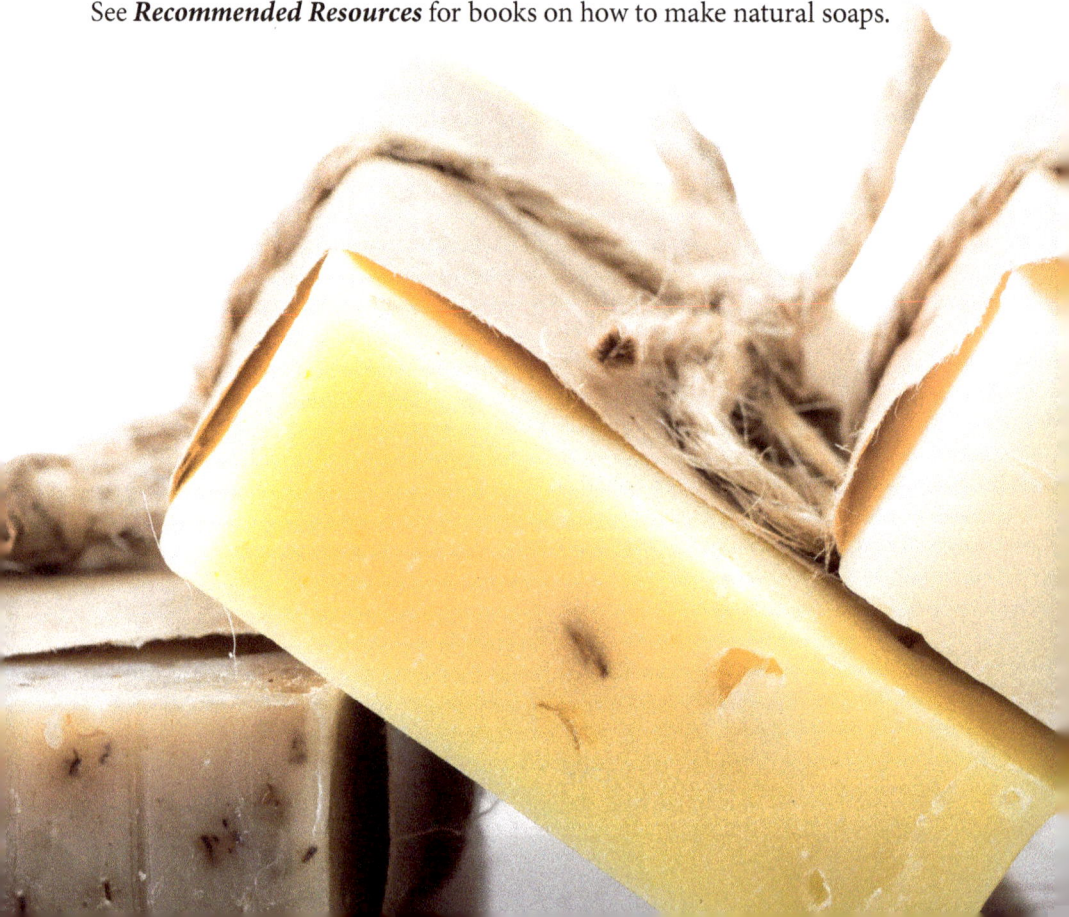

Only since the fourth century did the mixture of animal fat and ashes (lye) become a washing material for the body and clothes. For Ancient Israel, *ahala* was used as a cleanser. The exact definition of *ahala* is unclear, but it may refer to either a specific plant with roots that are rich in soda and alkaline, or perhaps all plants rich in soda and alkaline. The production of soap typically needs an alkaline solution.

One plant that *ahala* has been identified with is soapwort (*Saponaria officinalis*), also commonly called wild sweet William. The saponin found in the roots of soapwort produce a lather when in contact with water. One perfumed soap powder recipe from ancient Israel included *ahala*, myrtle, violet, frankincense powder and *kruspa de jasmine*. The latter was sesame residue soaked with jasmine roses and then dried and pulverized. (20:372; 16)

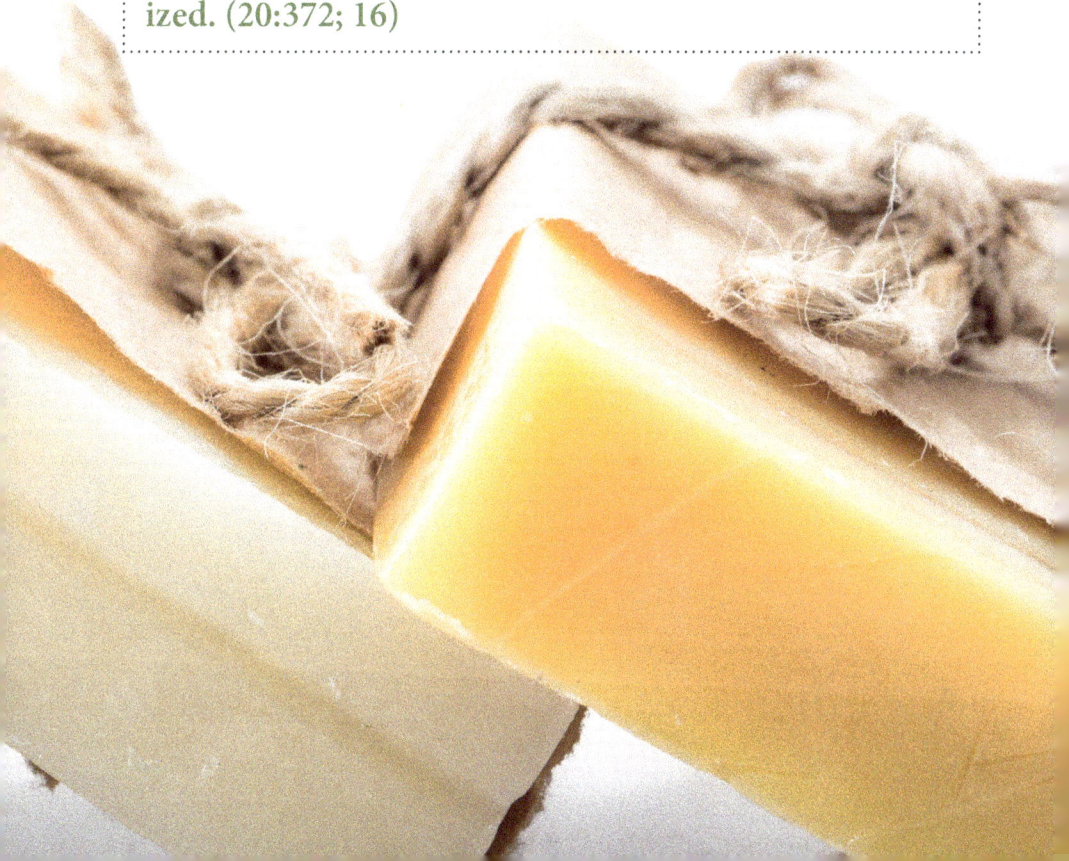

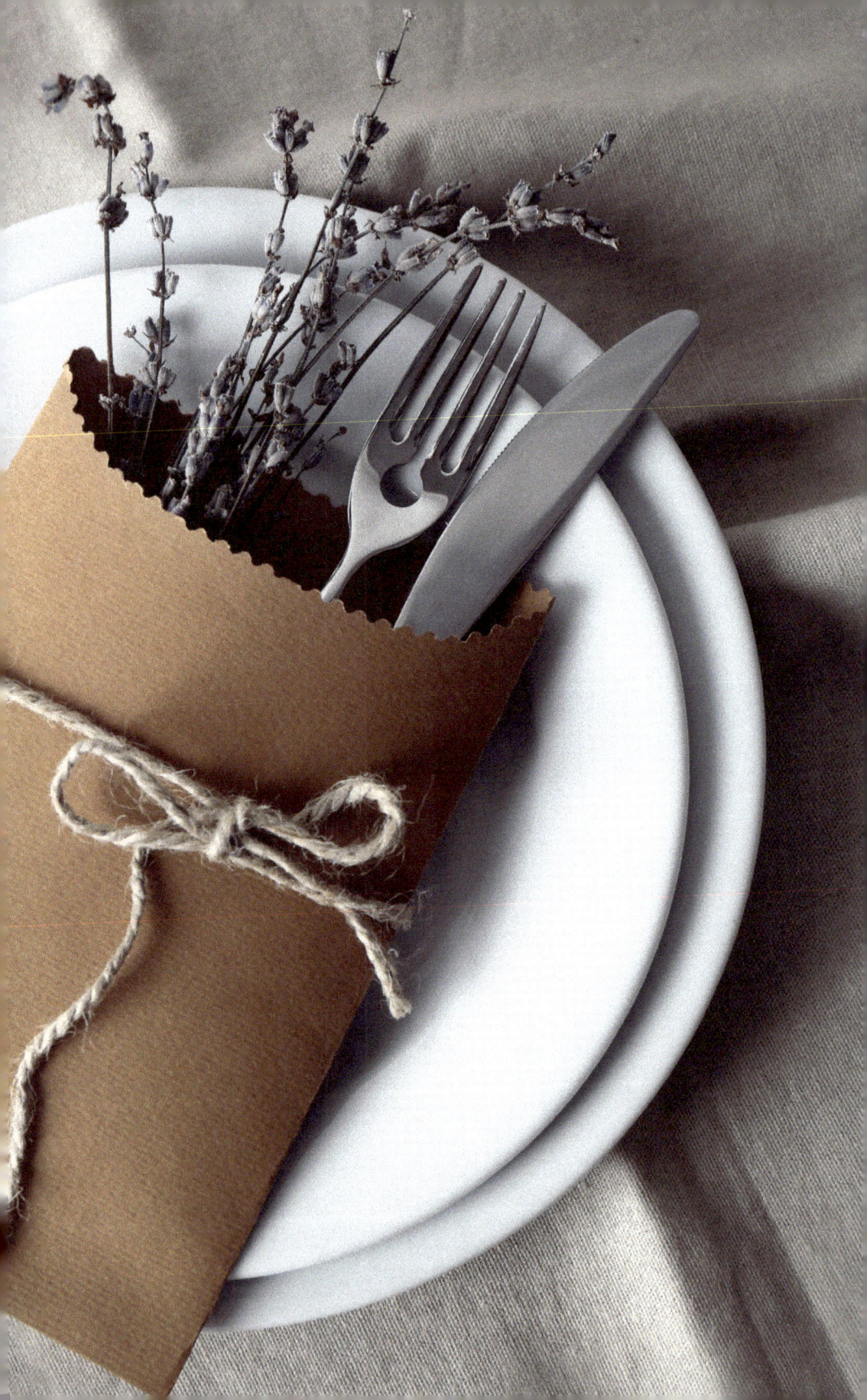

Household

Be creative with herbs in the day-to-day! Make the most of the plant parts, even adding them to the compost pile after they are spent. Here are some suggestions for inspiration.

Cleaning

- Infuse disinfecting herbs such as rosemary or lavender into white vinegar for a homemade cleaning solution. Add orange or lemon peels for extra fragrance and cleaning power. Add a few tablespoons of liquid soap for suds.

Freshening

- Place sprigs of lavender or other aromatic herbs in closets and dresser drawers to keep clothes and linens smelling fresh.

- Pillows or sachets filled with dried, fragrant herbs are another way to enjoy herbal scents. Fabric sachets can be put in the dryer with the laundry. You can also use them as coasters for hot beverages or the tea pot. They also become unique gifts and favors. Make your own sachets from light-weight cotton or other suitable fabric. Tie with a ribbon or sew closed.

  Note: Sachets lose their fragrance after a few months. They can be emptied and refilled.

- Dried herbs can become homemade potpourri. You can also add dried citrus peels, cinnamon sticks, whole spices or any fragrant flowers. To ensure the potpourri is completely dry and will not mold, spread materials on a wax-covered baking sheet and bake at 200°F for a few hours.

- During the winter, pinecones, rosemary and cinnamon sticks may be mixed into fireplace kindling to produce a cozy incense.

- Simmer fragrant herbs, spices and/or fruits on the stove to fill the house with a pleasant aroma.

Mary then took about a pint of pure nard, an expensive perfume; she poured it on Jesus' feet and wiped his feet with her hair. And the house was filled with the fragrance of the perfume. John 12:3

Cheering

- Fresh herb bouquets are colorful and fragrant. Add vases of bright wildflowers with green, aromatic foliage to the dinner table or around the house.

- Dried herb bouquets are also beautiful and sweet-smelling, and they last longer. Be sure to hang the herbs to dry completely before piecing together an arrangement.

- Consider featuring herbs at a dinner party or other event for a rustic theme. Herbs may be incorporated into place settings, décor and favors.

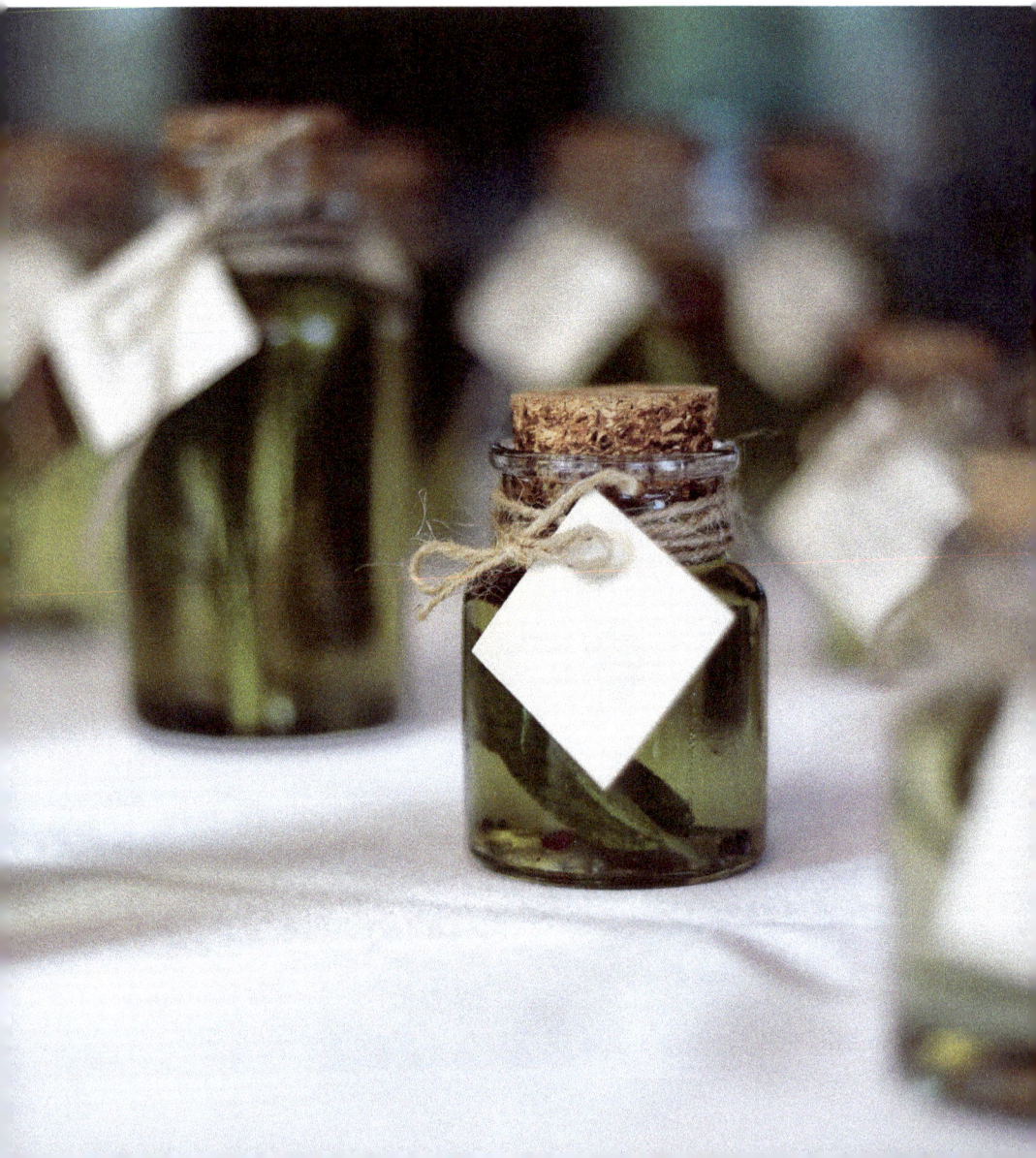

Medicine

Dear friend, I pray that you may enjoy good health and that all may go well with you, even as your soul is getting along well. 3 John 1:2

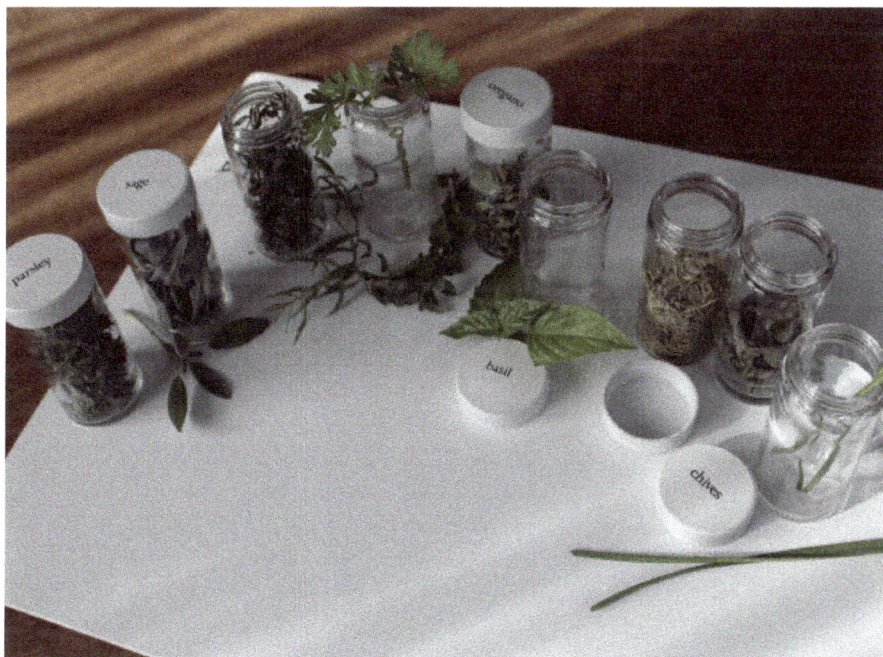

The next few pages contain the most common ways to use plants from your herb garden as medicine. Be sure to use all the safety measures outlined in this book. Many herbs are safe in culinary amounts but require more caution in medicinal amounts.

If you consult other sources, you may notice that instructions vary. To one herb crafter, a "decoction" means this, and to another it means that. Additional terminology and products also exist. This confirms that there are not set standards in the field, but it also means there is some flexibility. Just remember that it is always best to err on the side of caution.

Caution: If planning to ingest an herbal remedy, be sure use the correct part of the plant. Some plant parts are toxic.

Teas

Brewing a tea is the most common method for using herbs to boost health. The chemical compositions of herbal teas vary depending on the plants chosen. Though herbal teas have lower concentrations of antioxidants than green, black, white and oolong teas, they are beneficial for their own reasons. Some herbal teas have been known to fight the common cold or promote restful sleep, for some examples. (7)

The most common form of herbal tea is called an **infusion.** It is made by infusing dried plant material (herb leaves, flowers and berries) into hot water. Another form of herbal tea is called a **decoction.** Typically, this is when hard, dense materials need to be infused, such as seeds, roots or stems, which are simmered for up to an hour. More delicate materials are not ideal for decoctions. As a result of lengthy steeping, decoctions are stronger than infusions and not as palatable.

Infusion: Use one teaspoon of dried herb per cup of hot water. Steep for 10-20 minutes as desired, covered. Refrigerate if kept more than a few hours.

Decoction: Use one teaspoon of dried herb per cup of water. Bring to a boil and simmer for 40-60 minutes, covered. Refrigerate if kept more than a few hours.

Notes:

If using fresh herbs, double the amount.

If both an infusion and decoction are needed, make the decoction first with the hearty materials and add the delicate materials for the last 20 minutes.

*A cloth can be soaked in an herbal tea and applied to the body as a remedy. This is called a **fomentation** or a **compress.** Both hot or cold applications may be used as desired.*

See **Recommended Resources** for a book about crafting your own teas.

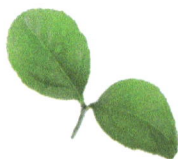

Herbal and botanical teas are caffeine-free. The reason other teas are caffeinated is because they all come from the plant *Camellia sinensis.* Whether white, green, oolong or black, the way tea leaves are processed determines what kind of tea results.

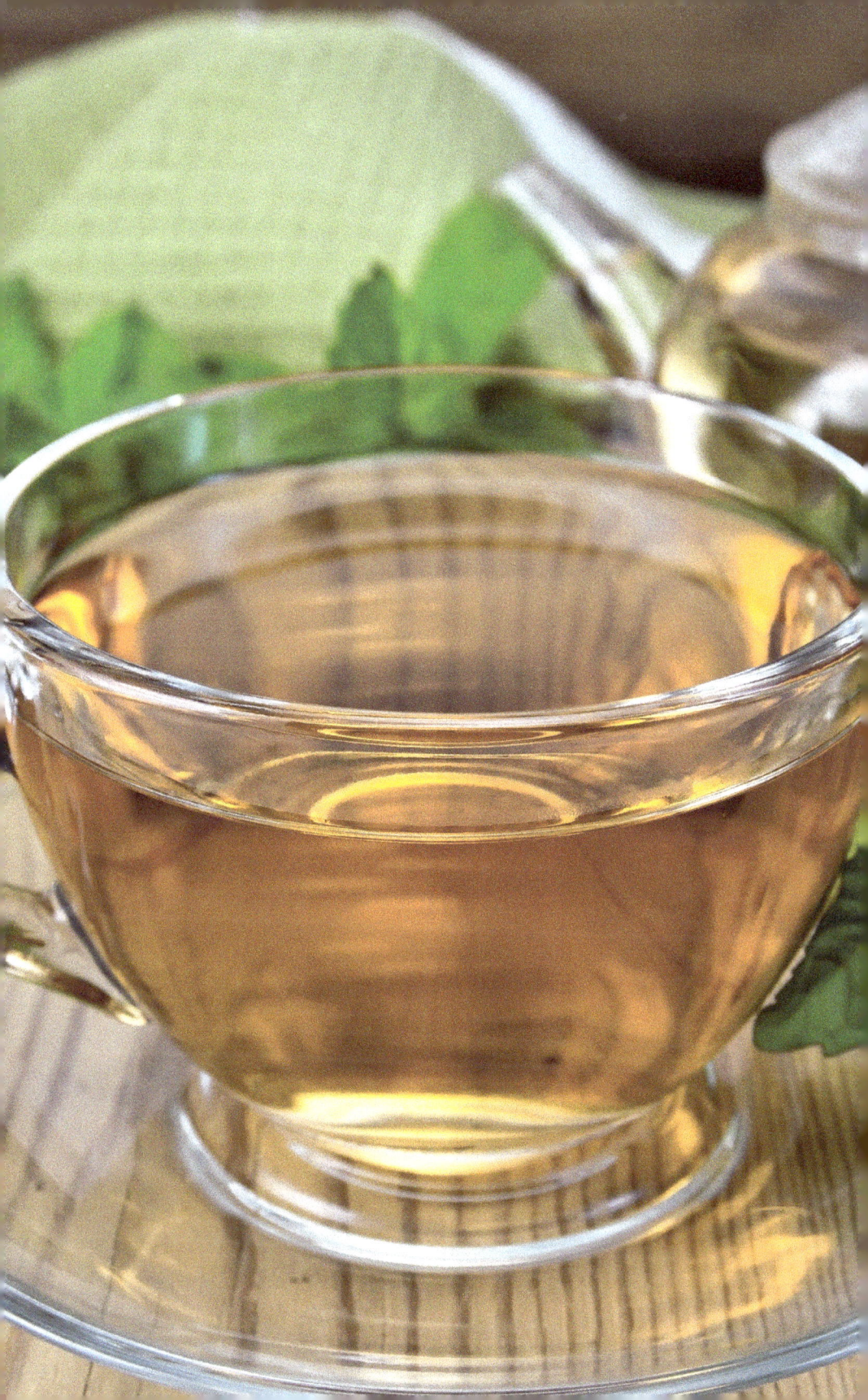

Tinctures

When many people think of herbal remedies, an image comes to mind of small, copper-colored bottles with droppers. These are called **tinctures,** or **extracts.** Tinctures are alcohol extracts of fresh or dried herbs.

Notice in this case, an infusion of herbs into alcohol is referred to as an *extract.* The word extract means to draw out. Alcohol draws out the constituents from the herb matter. Extracts are made the same way as infusions, but chopping and crushing the herbs boosts the extraction process.

To prepare a tincture, chop the desired fresh herbs or grind dried ones and place them in a glass jar. Cover the plant material with vodka or pure grain alcohol using a 1-1 plant to alcohol ratio. (1-4 for dried herbs.) Seal and place in a dark location, shaking a little every 2-3 days. After 4-6 weeks, strain the alcohol with cheesecloth and store in tincture bottles away from heat or sunlight. Discard after two years.

Note: Personally, I veer away from tinctures because of their potency and the many variables to consider. I have not had an occasion to make or use a tincture myself since other remedies have sufficed.

Dosage for Adults

In the field of herbal medicine, a commonly recommended tincture dose for an adult is thirty drops, three times a day. Nevertheless, only take a medicinal dose of an herbal remedy if you are confident that it is safe. (See **How to Use Herbs Safely**)

For acute problems, herbal remedies are usually taken only for the short duration of the condition. In this way, stronger doses may still be safe. However, for chronic conditions, experts suggest smaller doses along with breaks every few weeks to clear accumulation of constituents in the body.

Active constituents are the chemicals within herbs that have a physiological activity on the body. Their actions in the body are referred to as their pharmacology.

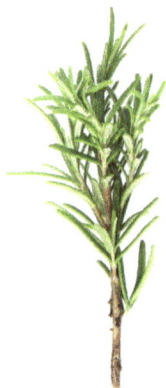

Dosage for Children

Dónal O'Mathúna, PhD, and Walt Larimore, MD, authors of *Alternative Medicine: The Christian Handbook*, do not recommend children taking herbal remedies unless proven safe. Currently, there is very limited information available.

If giving a proven herbal remedy to a child, information derived from the American College of Healthcare Sciences (ACHS) recommends limiting the dose using Clark's Rule and only for a short duration. **Clark's Rule** is a medical term that refers to calculating the amount of medicine for children aged 2-17. Take the child's weight divided by 150 to get the fraction dose. For example, a 50-pound child would take 1/3 of the recommended adult dose.

If an alcohol-free tincture is desired for any reason, such as to give to a child, vegetable glycerin can be used instead. Glycerin tastes sweet and is often made from coconut oil or vegetable oil. A glycerin extract is called a **glycerite.** Discard glycerites after six months.

Tip: Glycerites can also be used in teas or drizzled over desserts.

Poultices

A **poultice** is a warmed paste of organic materials that is applied to an affected area of the body. Poultices are meant to reduce aches and pains or allieviate bruises and wounds. If using chemically hot herbs, such as oregano, the poultice should not be warmed. It may result in a burning sensation to the skin.

To make an herbal poultice, wrap chopped herb matter in a cotton cloth. Soak in warm water to heat. Poultices can be reheated and reapplied 2-3 times. Discard after one day.

Poultices were in use in Bible times. Moist materials were spread over a wound or pain. Isaiah had a poultice of figs made for King Hezekiah to heal a boil. (2 Kings 20:7) Olive oil was usually involved in wound care (Isa. 1:6; Luke 10:34), sometimes as oil fomenting (20:238).

Ointments, Balms and Salves

In general, anti-bacterial **ointments** are products that protect and heal open wounds or scratches. **Balms** are used for soothing the skin, such as lip balms. **Salves** usually have a softer consistency than balms. Otherwise, these three terms are used interchangeably.

For a simple recipe, measure one cup of pure plant oil or infused oil into a small saucepan. Add two tablespoons (1 oz.) of beeswax. Once ingredients have combined, pour into containers, such as shallow tins. Let cool. The product will set. Discard after one month, or six months if refrigerated.

Note: *Alternatively, this product can be made into a lotion or cream before it sets. Slowly add water or an herbal tea. Use a blender to thicken.*
(See **Lotions and Creams**.)

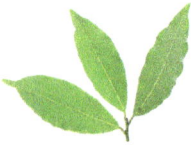

Salves were in use in Bible times.
Their bases were tallow and wax.

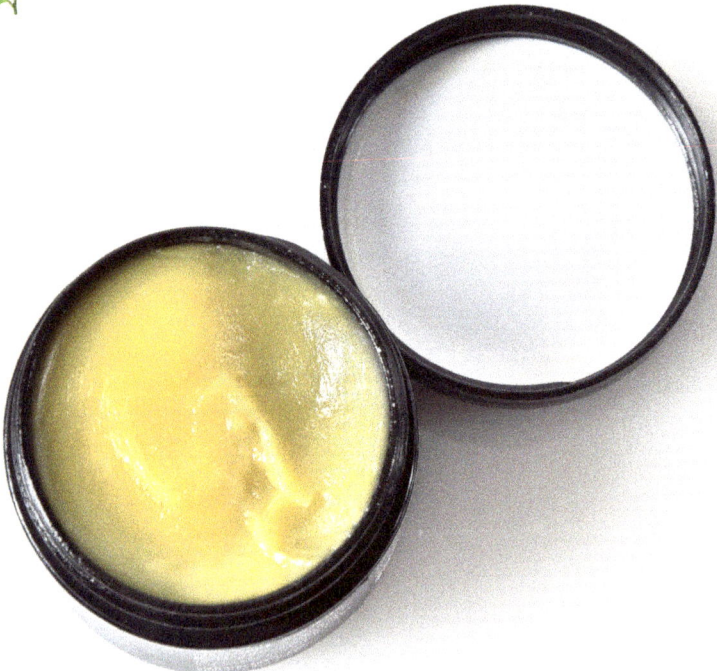

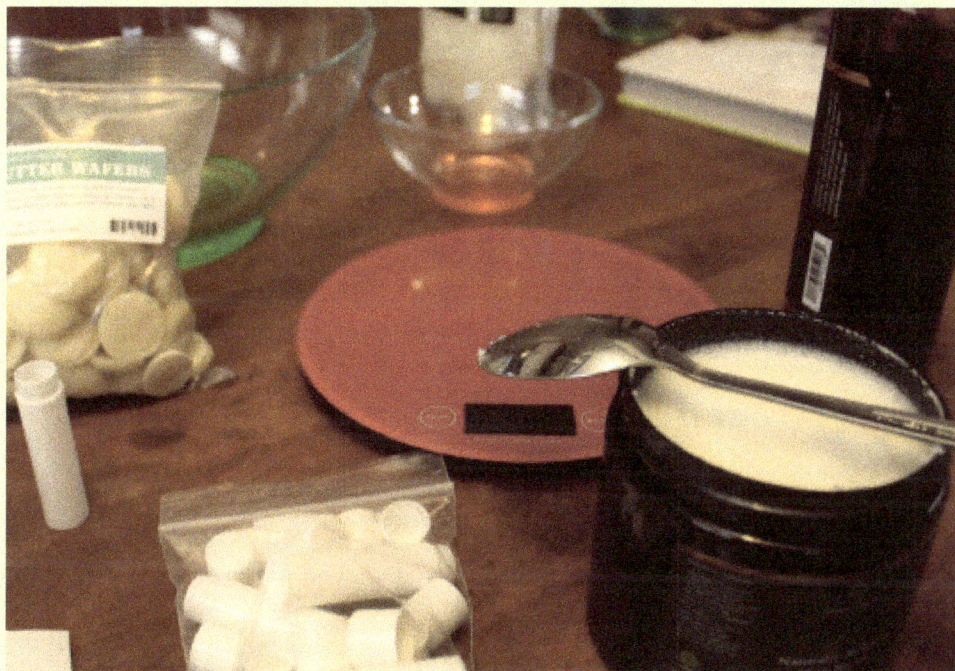

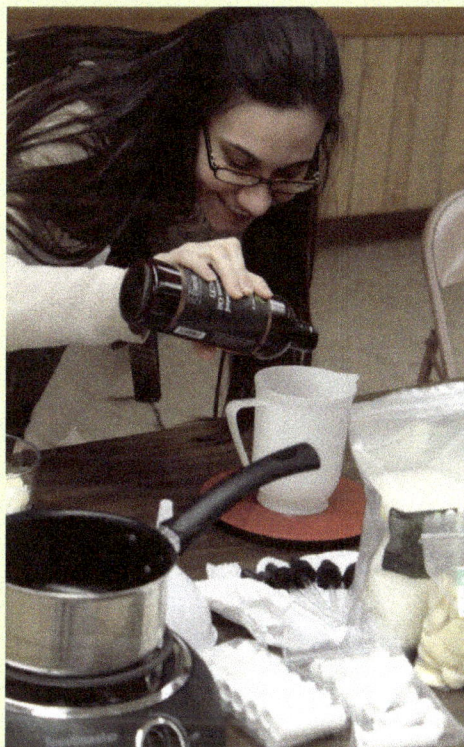

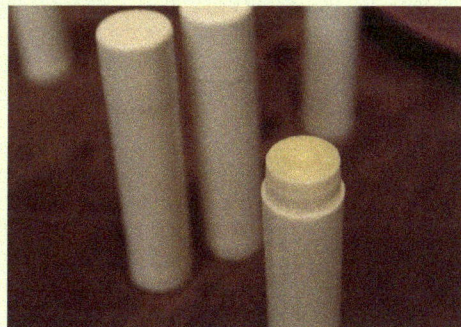

The Best Lip Balm

1 oz. beeswax
1 oz. coconut oil (infused as desired)
½ oz. shea butter
½ oz. cocoa butter

Gently melt ingredients together using a double boiler. When wax is melted, pour into lip balm tubes and let cool. *Makes 20.*

Common Medicinal Herbs

Aloe

The gel of Aloe vera leaves soothes minor burns and skin sores.

Calendula

Facilitates wound healing and reduces inflammation.

Chamomile

Used for calming nerves and bringing a restful sleep.

Comfrey

Believed to be effective for bruising and external wounds and sores.

Caution: Comfrey contains compounds that are toxic to the liver and can cause liver cancer. Do not ingest.

Echinacea

Stimulates the immune system, reducing cold and flu symptoms.

Feverfew

Used to help prevent migraines but does not reduce a fever.

Garlic

A germ killer, inhibiting various fungi, bacteria and yeasts; lowers cholesterol; believed to reduce blood pressure.

Ginger

Used to abate nausea and vomiting.

Lavender

Soothing in skincare products; may reduce anxiety and improve sleep.

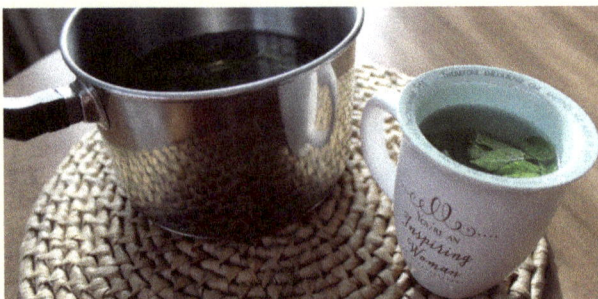

Mint

Used to allay cold and flu symptoms.

Mullein

Used to reduce congestion and to relive coughs and sore throats.

Nettles

Shown to be effective in relieving symptoms of osteoarthritis and prostate gland enlargement.

Oregano

Settles the stomach, relieves digestion and eases a cough.

Parsley

A breath freshener. In tea, parsley is an antihistamine that can relieve hay fever and hives.

Rosemary

Relaxes muscles, including in the digestive tract and uterus – relieving digestive issues and menstrual cramping.

Sage

In tea, helps soothe sore throats.

Tarragon

Can relieve minor mouth and toothache pain.

Thyme

Antibacterial and antifungal; can loosen phlegm, relieve coughs and aid digestion.

Valerian

Used to calm nerves.

Yarrow

Used for treating minor wounds.

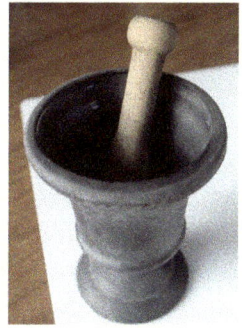

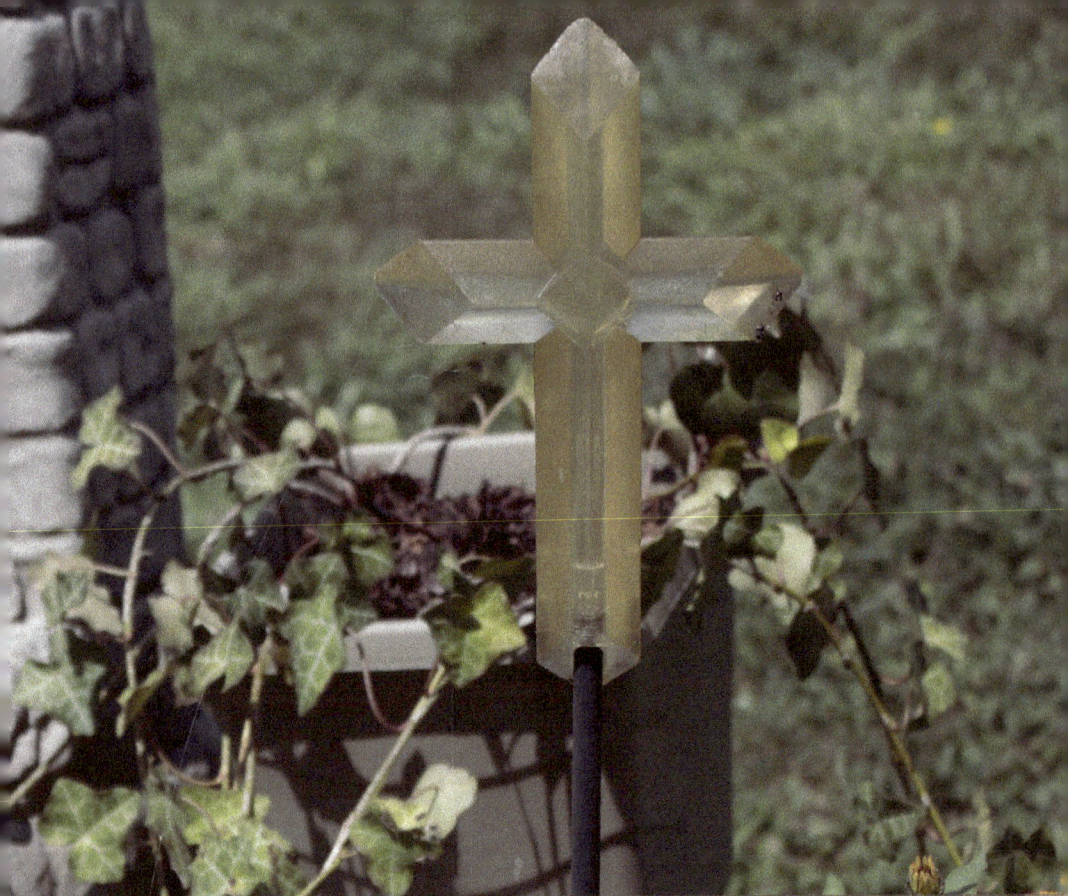

Herbs *and* Oils *of the* Bible

They also made the sacred anointing oil and the pure,
fragrant incense - the work of a perfumer. Exod. 37:29

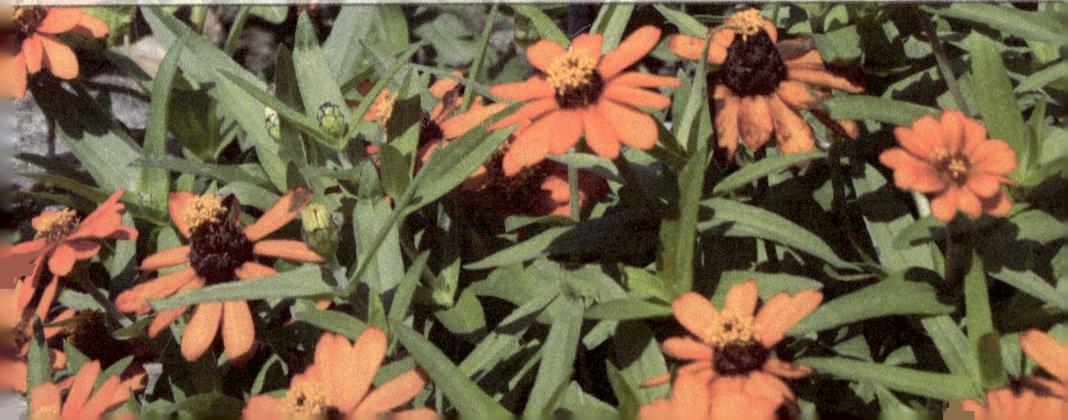

Marketing Schemes

Christians are often drawn to advertisements for "herbs of the Bible" or "oils of the Bible." Bible students know that the more they understand the culture of Bible times, the more the Scriptures will come to life. Furthermore, we might also reason that if God's provisions in the land flowing with milk and honey were suitable for the Hebrews, they are likely still healthful choices for us today.

Although a study of food, plant life or olive oil in Bible times can offer valuable insights, Christians should be aware of marketing that is targeted specifically for them. Consumers may be lured into purchasing unnecessary or expensive products promoted as biblical but that are *not* from the Bible. Or worse, they may be ensnared by herbalism or other forms of energy medicine.

The truth is that the Bible mentions 128 plants that were part of everyday life in ancient Israel, but these cannot all be identified with certainty today. According to the late, renowned botanist James Duke, the Bible's authors meant the plant references to be historical and not a guide for modern botanists. Both authors and translators of the Scriptures were familiar with agriculture more than botany. Early translators did not have access to good botanical research, and they were forced to make guesses. (5:18-20)

Today, there are still many difficulties correlating modern botanical species with plants of the Bible. Both botanical and biblical scholars disagree amongst themselves about the origins of the plants in the Scriptures. Essentially, they are still forced to make guesses. (5:8-9) For example, there are about seventeen different plants, herbs, sap residues and gum resins that might have been the balm of Gilead. (5:20)

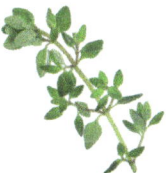

The balm of Gilead appears to have been applied in wound care in ancient Israel. (Jer. 8:22)

Duke may have said it best when he noted that the past biblical authors, prophets and theologians were "more concerned with our souls than our botany." (5:9) They had the right idea.

Similarly, the fragrant oils mentioned in the Scriptures are also not the concentrated, essential oil products we find on the market today. Many advertisements for essential oils claim that the products are mentioned in the Bible hundreds of times. However, do not be deceived. The real oils of the Bible were not akin to distilled, standardized, commercial essential oils. When specific spices are named in the Scriptures, aromatic perfumes were often meant. Plant oils were infused with spices to create perfumes. (20:370) For the Hebrews, the base oil was often olive oil, a top commodity of Israel.

In fact, when the word "oil" is mentioned in Scripture, it is usually referring to olive oil. The most common word for oil in the Old Testament, *shemen*, occurs 192 times. It refers to olive oil the majority of the time. The Greek word that corresponds to *shemen* in the New Testament is *elaion*. The eleven times that it is used refers exclusively to olive oil.

Furthermore, the precious and costly perfumes known to the ancient Hebrews were also not used in excess the way that some essential oil companies would have consumers use their products today. Perfumes were often saved for special purposes, such as worship or burial.

Consider when Judas grumbled: "Why wasn't this perfume sold and the money given to the poor?" Mary had just broken her jar of pure nard to pour over Jesus' feet. Judas went on, "It was worth a year's wages." (John 12:5)

Often herb and essential oil marketing to Christians even takes Scripture verses out of context. One common example is the quoting the last part of Revelation 22:2: "...*And the leaves of the tree are for the healing of the nations.*" This verse is not referring to the healing properties of oils from leaves of trees found on the earth today. It is from a prophetic passage describing the future New Jerusalem. The special tree will be in heaven, and the way it will function is unknown.

Therefore, the claim that a product is from the Bible may be very misleading. A consumer might be more likely to believe the product is safe in ways that it is not. Although certain common names of herbs do appear in the Scriptures, safety measures should always be taken for all herbs, for their products and for their essential oils. (See **How to Use Herbs Safely**)

Your plants are an orchard of pomegranates with
choice fruits, with henna and nard, nard and saffron,
calamus and cinnamon, with every kind of incense
tree, with myrrh and aloes and all the finest spices.
Song 4:13-14

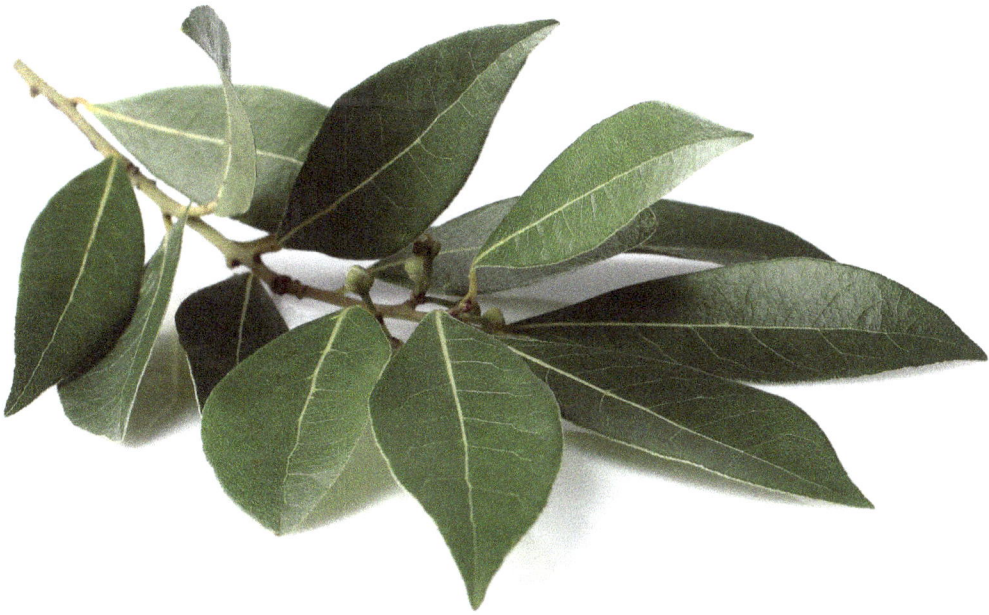

Incense and perfumes found in the Bible are not limited to an association with the Jewish or Christian faiths. Many of the same aromatic herbs were also used in pagan worship of false gods throughout the ancient world. Various herbal preparations continue to be used today for similar purposes.

*For the Lord your God is bringing you into a good land – a land with
brooks, streams, and deep springs gushing out into the valleys and
hills; a land with wheat and barley, vines and fig trees, pomegranates,
olive oil and honey; a land where bread will not be scarce and you will
lack nothing; a land where the rocks are iron and you can dig copper
out of the hills. Deut. 8:7-9*

The Land Flowing with Milk and Honey

The *land flowing with milk and honey* (Exod. 3:17) described a grazing land
not overly cultivated. There were plenty of cattle for milk and abundant wildflowers for bees to produce honey. Several kinds of fruit trees grew in Israel that
could also produce products as sweet as a bee's honey, such as date honey. (26:6,
72)

In this promised, holy land, the Israelites knew cedars, sycamore trees, and
wild grasses and herbs. The bitter herbs used in their Passover meals could have
been chicory, sea holly (26:53), mallows, radishes, dandelions and others. (5:26;
Exod. 12:8) Israelites were familiar with "cucumbers, melons, leeks, onions, and
garlic." (Num. 11:5) They culti-
vated the Seven Species – wheat,
barley, grapes, figs, olives, pomegranates and dates. (26:7)

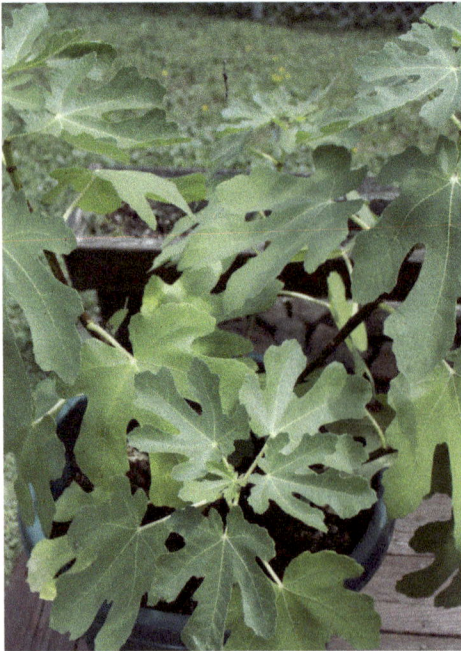

On their tables were almonds
and capers, lentils and chickpeas,
beans and eggs. Apples, apricots
and other fruits and nuts appeared
after having been introduced
through trade. Meats were preserved with salt and spices. Breads
were sometimes baked with herbs.
They flavored their dishes with "all
the fine spices," even roses. (26:56)
Wines were sweetened by adding
raisins, honey or other fruit juice.
Spiced wines may have been infused with cardamom and saffron.
(26:35)

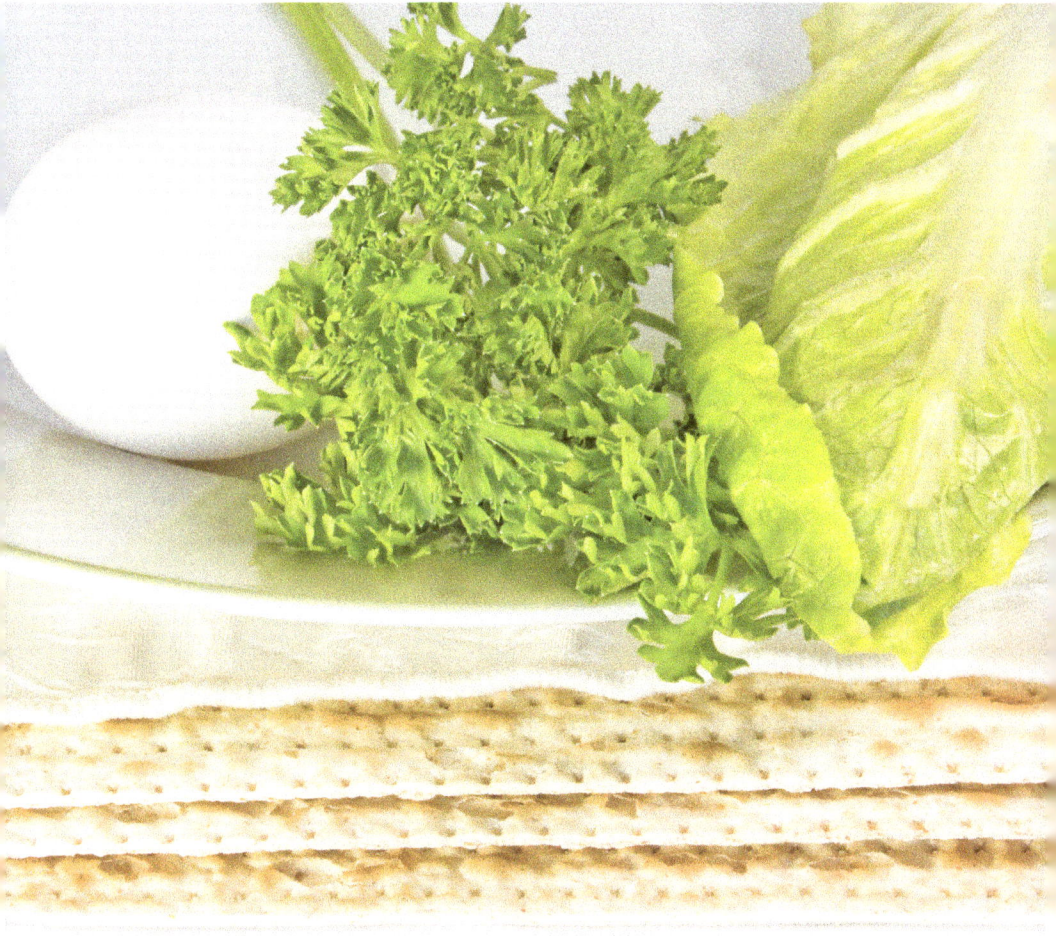

Many spices mentioned in the Bible were never grown in the Middle East but were imported, such as spikenard, myrrh, galbanum and cinnamon. (5:18)

The berries of the sumaq plant of the Holy Land (*Rhus coriaria*) were ground into a reddish-brown powder that served the same purposes in cooking as we use lemon, which was unavailable. (26:77)

Common Herbs and Spices in New Testament Times

Aloes

The aloes of the Bible are most likely derived from the sap of the eaglewood tree (*Aquilaria agallocha*), which is native to India. (The American aloe plant is a succulent.) These aloes retain their fragrance for years. The feature would have been ideal since tombs were re-opened to bury more family members.

...Nicodemus brought a mixture of myrrh and aloes, about seventy-five pounds. Taking Jesus' body, the two of them wrapped it, with the spices, in strips of linen. This was in accordance with Jewish burial customs. John 19:39-40

Anise

The seeds of the anise plant were sprinkled on bread just before baking. In the fall, wild anise plants perfumed the air of Israel's mountains with a spicy-sweet licorice aroma.

Bay tree (Laurel)

The oil of bay trees was used in perfumes.

Cinnamon

The cinnamon tree migrated to Israel from China. Cinnamon was found in the Holy Incense of the Tabernacle. It also found its way into other perfumes in Bible times. Says the adulterous woman of Proverbs 7, "I have perfumed my bed with myrrh, aloes and cinnamon." (Prov. 7:17)

Cumin

Cumin is native to Israel. It was used to season meat.

Woe to you, teachers of the law and Pharisees, you hypocrites! You give a tenth of your spices – mint, dill and cumin. But you have neglected the more important matters of the law – justice, mercy and faithfulness. You should have practiced the latter, without neglecting the former. Matt. 23:23

Note: Black cumin is a different plant. It produces black seeds. To harvest black cumin seeds, they were threshed with sticks. Black cumin was sometimes mistranslated as "dill." (Isa. 28:27)

Coriander

Coriander is native to the Mediterranean region. It was introduced to Europe during Roman rule. Pliny the Elder reports that the best coriander came from Egypt. That may be why Moses was able to describe manna as "white like coriander seed," if in fact the name of the spice was not mistranslated.

The people of Israel called the bread manna. It was white like coriander seed and tasted like wafers made with honey. Exod. 16:31

Fragrant Cane (Calamus)

Sweet aromatic calamus was used as a perfume and for embalming. It smells like ginger. Calamus was also an ingredient in the Holy Anointing Oil recipe.

Take the following fine spices: 500 shekels of liquid myrrh, half as much (that is, 250 shekels) of fragrant cinnamon, 250 shekels of fragrant calamus, 500 shekels of cassia – all according to the sanctuary shekel – and a hin of olive oil. Exod. 30:23-24

Gall (Wormwood)

Gall is a bitter-tasting herb used in Scripture as a metaphor for bitterness.

He has filled me with bitter herbs and given me gall to drink. Lam. 3:15

Hyssop

Hyssop is native to the Holy Land. It can be found throughout Scripture symbolically associated with purity or cleansing. The hyssop branch was used to brush lamb's blood onto doorposts during the first Passover and was also given to Jesus the Lamb of God as a drink during His crucifixion. Hyssop was used to prepare the ashes of the Red Heifer and for the purification ceremony of lepers.

Cleanse me with hyssop, and I will be clean; wash me, and I will be whiter than snow. Ps. 51:7

Mint

Mint was used to season meat. It thrives along the Dan River and other streams. (Matt. 23:23)

Mustard

The mustard plant (*Sinapis alba*) produces tiny seeds just like in the parable. Mustard grows rampant and wild in the Holy Land. However, as it does not become the size of a tree, scholars have suggested that the shrub *Salvadora persica* was meant in the well-known parable instead.

Then Jesus asked, "What is the kingdom of God like? What shall I compare it to? It is like a mustard seed, which a man took and planted in his garden. It grew and became a tree, and the birds perched in its branches. Luke 13:18-19

Myrrh

Gold, frankincense and myrrh were the famous gifts brought to the Christ child by wise men from the east. Gold was a traditional tribute for a king. Frankincense was used in religious rituals and offerings. Myrrh anointed the dead for burial while symbolizing bitter tears. When gifted to the child, myrrh prefigured Jesus' death and indicated His humanity. The three gifts were appropriate for a king, a God and a man.

Both frankincense and myrrh are fragrant gum resins from trees, but myrrh oozes naturally whereas cuts are made for frankincense. Historically, hardened sap of myrrh was ground and added to perfumes, cosmetics, medicines and wines. Myrrh as a spice made low-quality wine more palatable.

On coming to the house, they saw the child with his mother Mary, and they bowed down and worshiped him. Then they opened their treasures and presented him with gifts of gold, frankincense and myrrh. Matt. 2:11

Nard (Spikenard)

Nard is a member of the valerian family. Its roots were used for perfume and as a sedative. The full name "Spikenard" comes from the spikes that shoot from the root. Mary used an expensive perfume of pure nard to anoint Jesus' feet. (John 12:3)

Rue (Fitch)

Rue is a shrub native to the Mediterranean regions. Luke tells us it was one of the garden herbs tithed by the Pharisees. (Luke 11:42)

Saffron

Saffron is produced by flowers in the crocus family. The plants were harvested for their yellow stigmas that were used in perfumes, cooking, medicine and dyes. Since only three stigmas can be harvested from each flower, the spice was costly and still is today. Saffron was also popular in ancient Persia during the time of Xerxes and could have been used in Esther's beauty treatments.

Before a young woman's turn came to go in to King Xerxes, she had to complete twelve months of beauty treatments prescribed for the women, six months with oil of myrrh and six with perfumes and cosmetics. Esth. 2:12

Sage

Sage is not mentioned in the Bible, but it is common in the Holy Land.

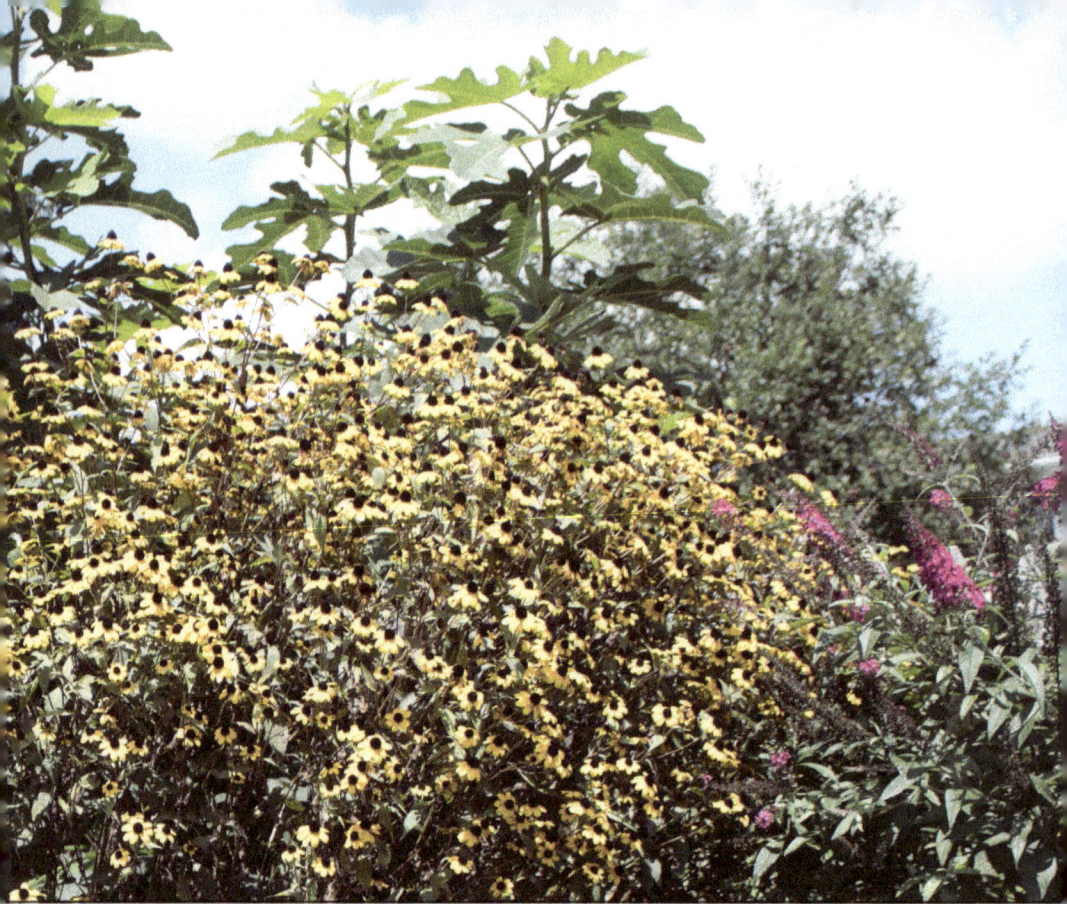

Relevant Herbs *at a* Glance

In addition to being used for food, beauty or medicine, herbs also add charm, fragrance and color to the garden. The following are some of the most popular herbs that appeared in this book.

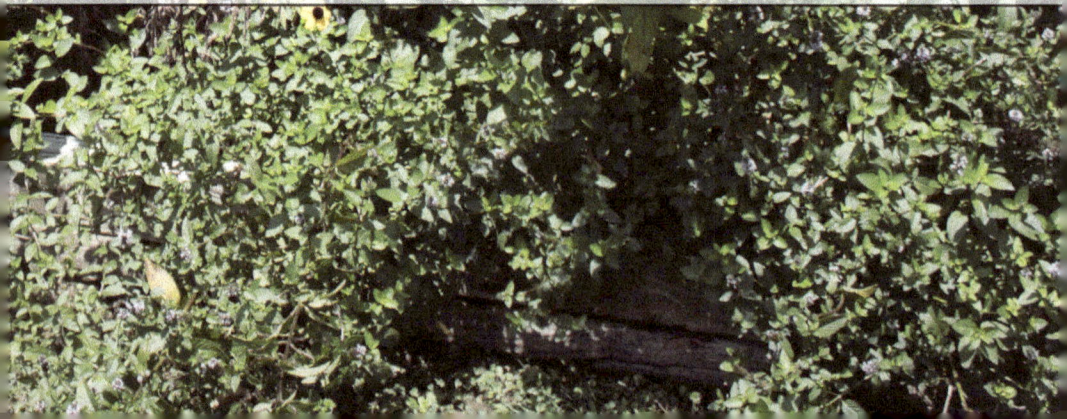

Aloe

Aloe barbadensis **(Aloe vera)**
Tender Perennial
Zones 9 and 10 (or as an indoor plant)

Aloe prefers sun but can tolerate shade. It does well enough in low-nutrient soil, but good drainage is required. Aloe is low maintenance. Infrequent waterings suffice. If leaf shoots are thin and firm, more water is needed to plump them. When the plant becomes crowded, divide it by rooting one of the offshoots formed near the base. Shake the mother plant from the pot and gently pull the offshoot away.

To harvest: Remove outer leaves first. New leaves grow from the center of the plant.

To use: Slice a leaf down the center and apply gel to burns, sunburn and skin sores.

Caution: Aloe vera is safe for topical use, but clinical tests do not support using it internally.

> A tender perennial will live year to year in warmer zones, but it will not survive in a cold climate.

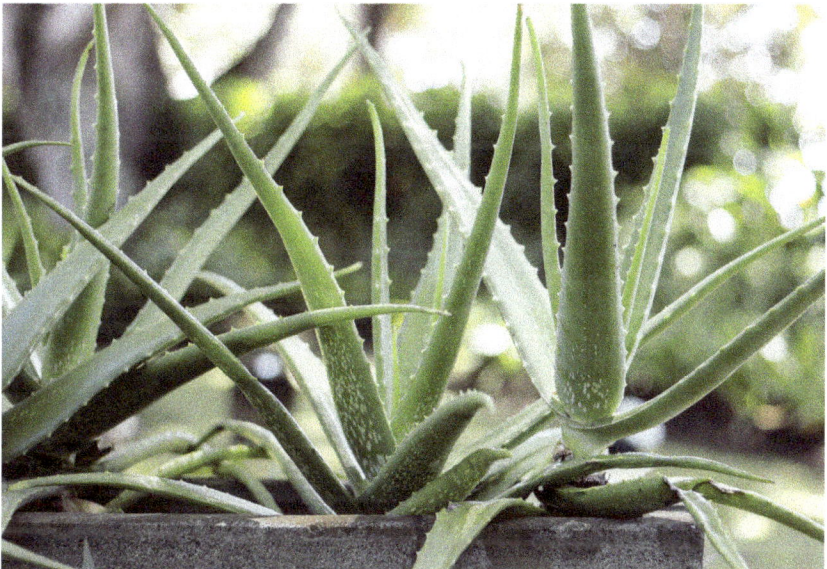

Angelica

Angelica archangelica
Biennial
Zones 4-9

Angelica prefers partial shade. It can grow in the sun if mulched. Space plants two feet apart as Angelica can grow up to eight feet tall. Soil should be average fertility. The plant can be susceptible to aphids, earwigs, leafminers and spider mites. It can also contract crown rot. Angelica will die after setting seeds. Therefore, remove flowers if you wish to prolong life.

Garden Splendor: Flowers look like Queen-Anne's lace. They bloom in June or July during the second year, sometimes the third.

Parts used: All parts can be used in cooking. Even the root is aromatic. The flavor of Angelica is like mild licorice.

To harvest: Gather leaves and stems before the plant flowers. Dig roots in early fall after the first year.

To use: Stems can be prepared like asparagus. They can also be stewed with fruits, minced in preserves or candied to sweeten desserts. Leaves can be used as flavoring for dishes.

Caution: Causes photosensitivity.

Partial Shade means 3-6 hours of sun, preferably morning or early afternoon sun. The terms *Partial Sun* and *Partial Shade* are used interchangeably.

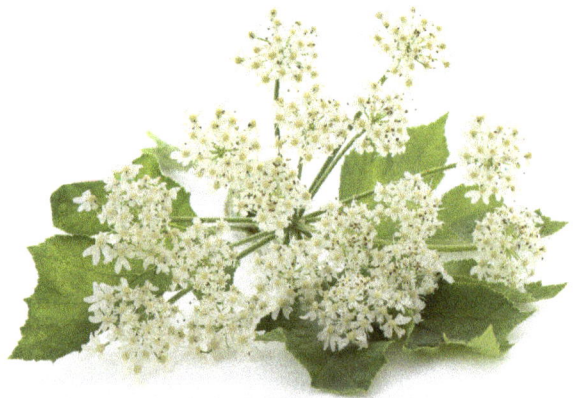

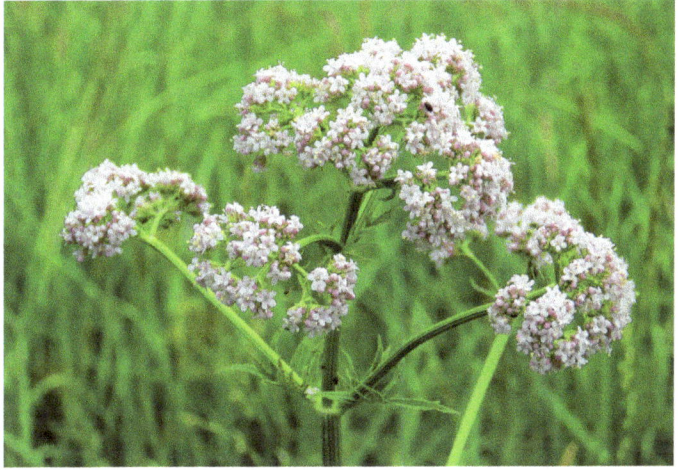

Anise

Pimpinella anisum
Annual

Anise will thrive in full sun. It does best in well-drained soil. Space seeds twelve inches apart in groups. Single plants may need to be staked to stay upright. Anise is pest and disease free.

Garden Splendor: Anise has ferny leaves and blooms that resemble Queen-Anne's lace. It has a spicy-sweet aroma.

Parts used: Leaves and seeds

To harvest: Cut stems at leaf node.

To use: Whole or ground seeds add sweetness to pastries, cakes and cookies. Leaves and seeds can both be used in salads. Leaves flavor chicken, fish and vegetables. Anise is recommended to aid in digestion or to soothe a cough. To do so, brew into a tea.

Caution: Anise may act like estrogen. Do not use if exposure to estrogen worsens a condition you may have.

Full Sun means at least six hours of direct sunlight.

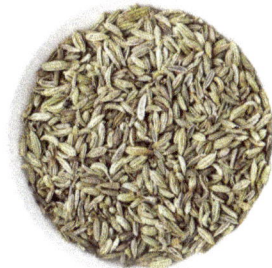

Basil

Ocimum basilicum
Annual

   Plant seeds/seedlings twelves inches apart. Basil prefers full sun and rich, moist, well-drained soil. Mulching again in midsummer will keep soil ideal. Pruning promotes leaf production. Pinch off the central stem tips frequently to encourage new growth. This produces a bushier plant rather than a tall, straggly one. Beware of some pests, such as aphids and slugs. Poorly drained soil and high humidity can cause disease. Basil is also sensitive to cold.

Garden Splendor: Basil is aromatic and pungent. It will grow spikes of tiny white, pink or purple florets. To preserve taste, do not let the flowers go to seed.

Parts used: Leaves

To harvest: Remove stems at leaf nodes or harvest individual leaves.

To use: Chop before adding to recipes. Basil is commonly used in Italian dishes. Leaves can also be infused into water for a refreshing drink, or into teas, vinegars and oils. Basil is believed to promote digestion.

Caution: Taking basil as a medicine long term may be unsafe. Basil extracts may also lower blood pressure and slow blood clotting.

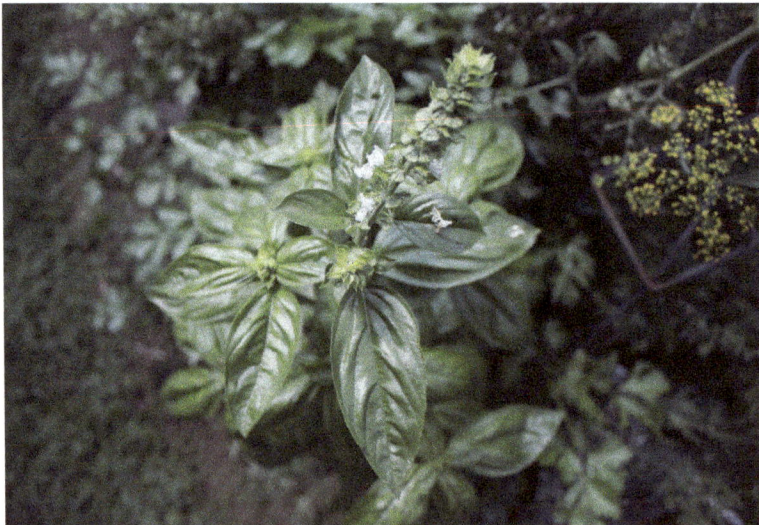

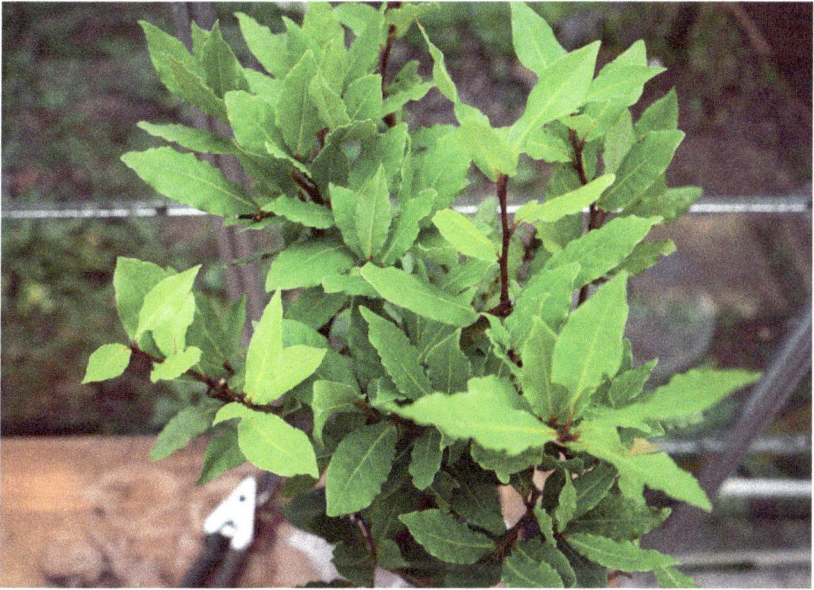

Bay

Laurus nobilis
Tender tree
Zones 8 and above (or in a container to be moved indoors during winter)

Wreaths of bay crowned the heads of royalty and victors in ancient Greece and Rome. Bay trees prefer full sun but can grow in light shade. They require moderately rich, well-drained soil. Bay can grow up to twenty feet tall. It is best to grow bay in a container in cold climates so it can overwinter indoors. Bay tolerates temperatures no lower than 20°F.

Parts used: Leaves

To harvest: Pinch off fresh leaves as needed.

To use: Bay leaves are added to soups, stews and sauces. They are especially popular in French dishes. Remove before serving. Bay can soothe the skin when added to a bath.

Caution: Bay leaves may slow the Central Nervous System. Cease medicinal use two weeks prior to a surgery. Bay leaves may also interfere with blood sugar control.

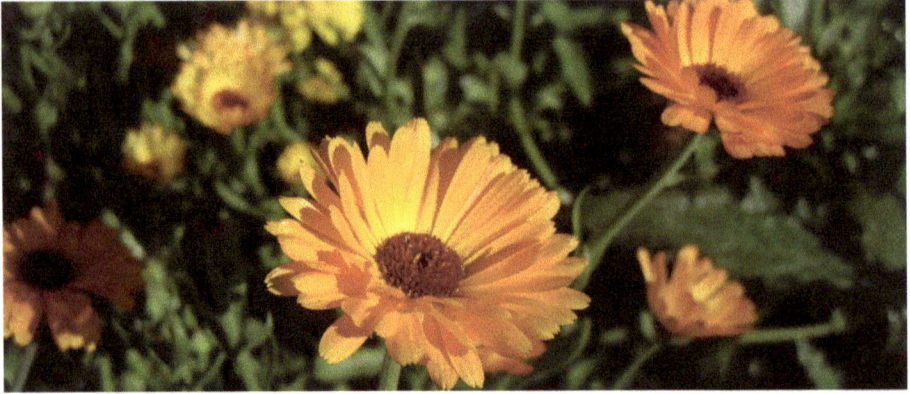

Calendula

Calendula officinalis
Annual

Calendula prefers full sun in the north (zones 5-6 and colder) and partial shade in the south (zones 7-9). Plant 8-10 inches apart in fertile, moist, well-drained soil. Calendula is susceptible to many diseases and has some pests.

Garden Splendor: Yellow or orange flowers brighten a garden. They close at dusk. The petals do not have a strong fragrance and are primarily used for color.

Parts used: Flowers

To harvest: Cut the stem at the joint that is closest to the flower you are harvesting.

To use: Add petals to salad or as a garnish for other dishes. Calendula flowers have been infused in massage oils and hair and skin products. Calendula can aid wound healing and reduce swelling and inflammation.

Caution: Beware of an allergy to the Asteraceae/Compositae family.

The description *offinalis* or *offinale* as the second term in a two-part botanical name denotes a use in medicine.

Chamomile

Chamaemelum nobile or Matricaria recutita
Perennial or Annual
Zones 5-9

The creeping perennial chamomile is often called Roman chamomile, *Chamaemelum nobile*. The upright species, *Matricaria recutita*, is called German chamomile. Both are used the same ways and are pest-free. Full sun to partial shade is needed, as well as good drainage. If starting from seed, space 12-18 inches apart in the spring.

Garden Splendor: Chamomile grows daisy-like flowers with white petals and yellow centers.

Parts used: Flowers

To harvest: Harvest flowers when the petals begin to turn back on the disk.

To use: Chamomile tea is a familiar remedy. It is used for calming nerves and bringing restful sleep, or for helping to relieve an upset stomach. Do not drink if you are allergic to ragweed or other daisy relatives. Make a compress from the tea to promote the healing of cuts, scrapes and mild burns.

Caution: People are more likely to experience allergic reactions to chamomile if they are allergic to related plants. Chamomile has interacted with some drugs and could interact with others. Therefore, speak with your doctor before medicinal use if you are taking any medications or sedatives.

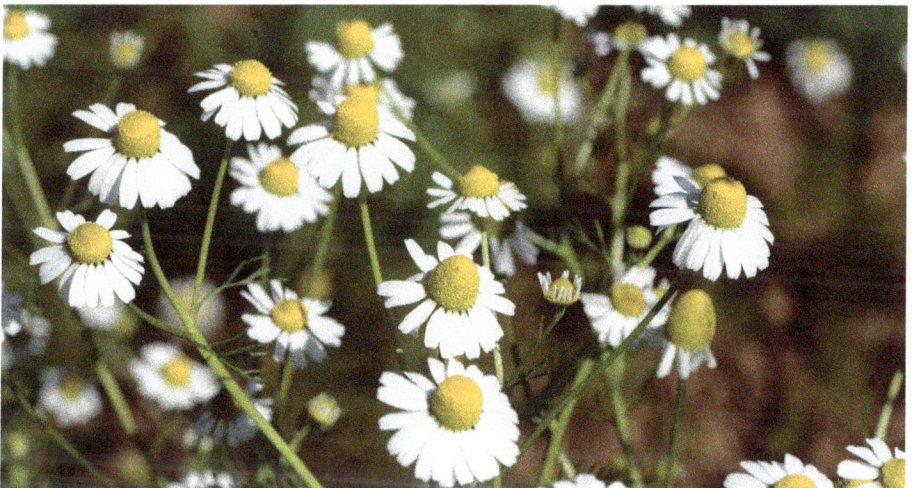

Chives

Allium schoenoprasum, chives
A. Tuberosum, garlic chives
Perennials
Zones 3-10

Chive seeds need darkness to germinate. Place plants in the garden 8-12 inches apart. They will do best with well-drained soil and compost. Chives need full sun to partial shade. Divide them every few years to prevent over-crowding by digging up the clump of roots and gently separating smaller clumps of bulbs. Chives become dormant in the winter. Garlic chives are especially hardy and survive winter even in very cold climates.

Garden Splendor: Chives will produce clusters of pink or purple florets. Their "leaves" are cylindrical. Garlic chives produce clusters of white flowers. Their "leaves" are flat.

Parts used: Leaves and flowers

To harvest: Wait until leaves are six inches tall. Cut about two inches above the soil. Cut back chives after they have flowered.

To use: Chives have an onion flavor. Garlic chives have a mild garlic flavor. Snip leaves into dishes. Add whole flowers into salads.

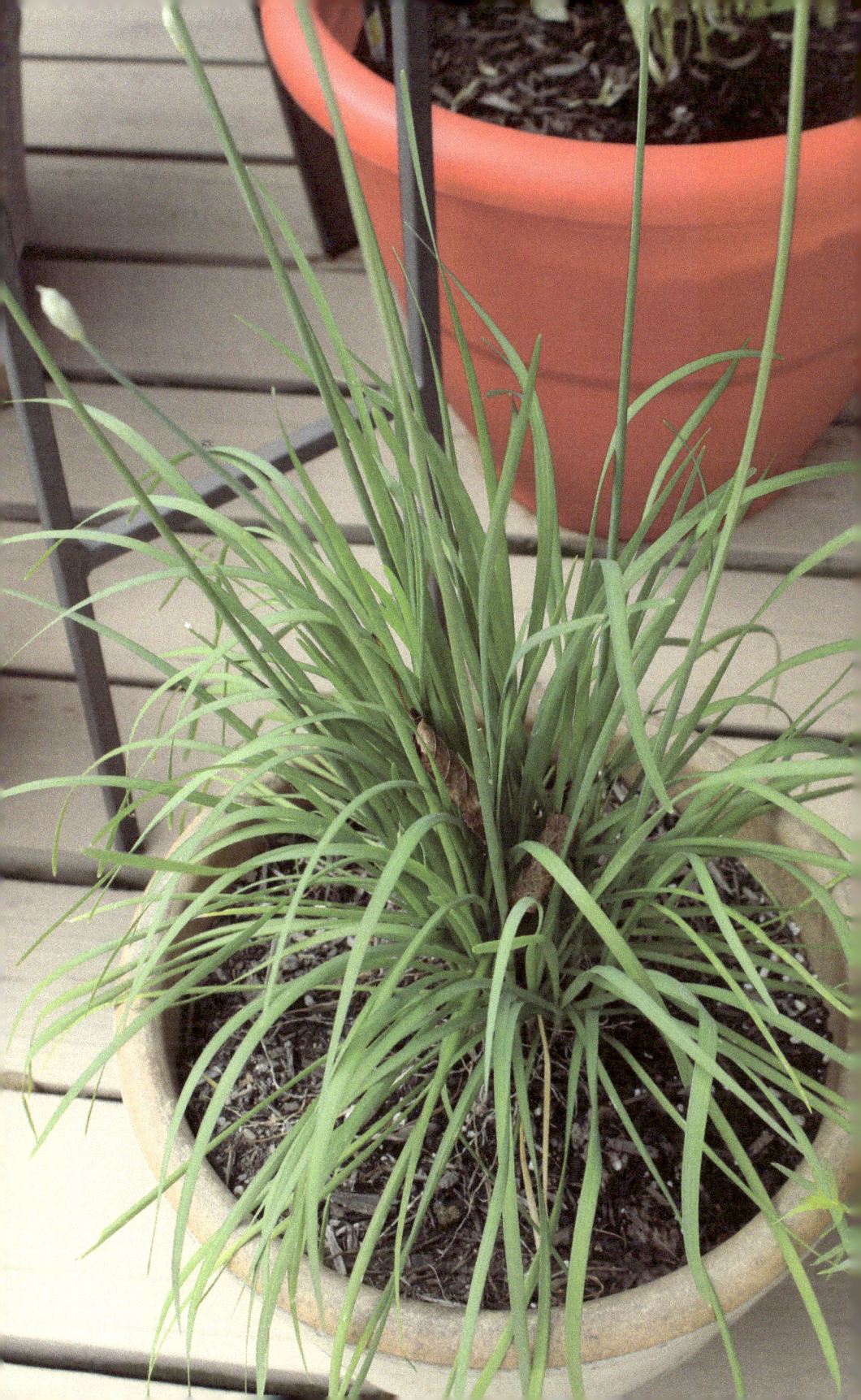

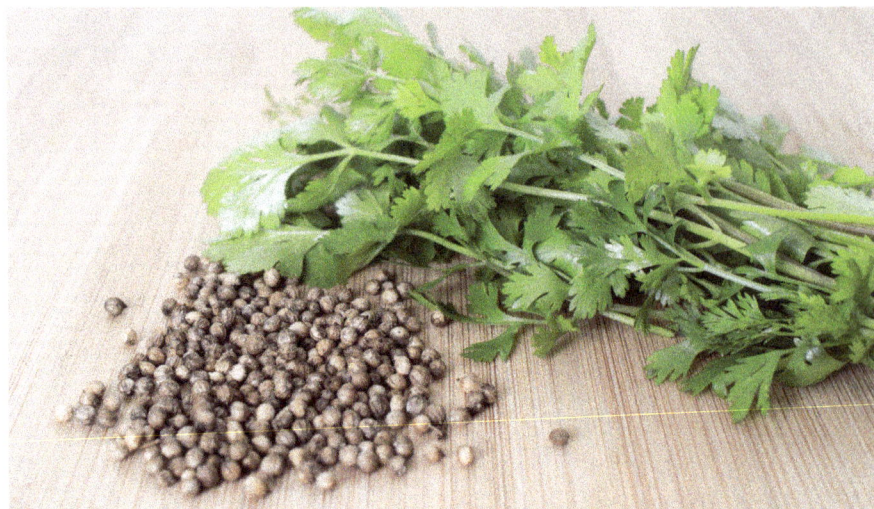

Coriander/Cilantro

Coriandrum sativum
Annual
Zones 3-8 (plant in the spring); Zones 9-11 (plant in the fall)

This herb will grow in moderately rich, light, well-drained soil. It likes full sun to partial shade. Sow the seed directly into the garden as it does not transplant well. Space plants 8-10 inches apart. This herb bolts quickly and easily. Cilantro may possibly survive a mild winter.

Parts used: Leaves and seeds

To harvest: Harvest leaves when plants are 5-6 inches tall. Cut stems at leaf nodes. Harvest seedheads (coriander seeds) when seeds are dry and fully ripe.

To use: Cilantro leaves are found in salsa and other tomato sauces. They can also be used in salads. Coriander seeds are used in curries and other dishes. Tea made with dried leaves or crushed seeds is used a mild digestive aid.

Caution: Used medicinally, coriander may lower blood sugar levels and decrease blood pressure.

Dandelion

Taraxacum officinale
Perennial

Dandelion is found growing in temperate regions of the world.

Parts used: All parts

To harvest: Snip parts needed or dig up by the root.

To use: Dandelion can be eaten raw in salads or blanched and used as a green. Flowers are used to make wine. Roasted roots are sometimes ground and brewed as coffee. Dandelion root has been used to help protect the liver, though studies are lacking. Dandelion may promote frequency of urination.

Caution: Side effects can include heartburn and diarrhea. Beware of allergies.

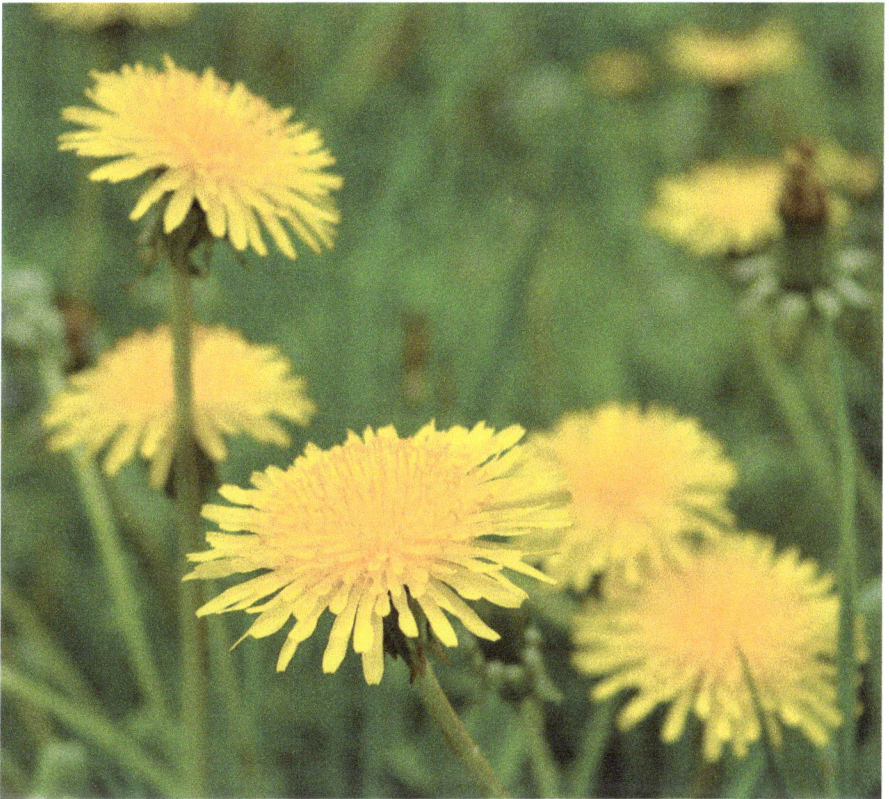

Dill

Anethum graveolens
Annual

Dill prefers full sun and moderately rich, moist, well-drained soil. Plant dill seeds 10-12 inches apart. Sow every three weeks to have a steady supply. Dill is generally pest and disease free. It will shoot up each year if the flowers go to seed.

Garden Splendor: Tiny umbrellas of yellow flowers bloom 3-4 months after sowing. They attract bees and other beneficial insects.

Parts used: Fronds (Leaves)

To harvest: Clip leaves close to the stem. Harvest seeds 2-3 weeks after they flower.

To use: Use leaves in salads or as a garnish. Add tangy flavor to many dishes, vinegars and oils. Of course, use in your favorite dill pickle recipe! Make a dill tea to soothe the stomach. Both leaves and seeds have been used for digestive aid.

Caution: Dill causes photosensitivity. Dill extract may lower blood sugar.

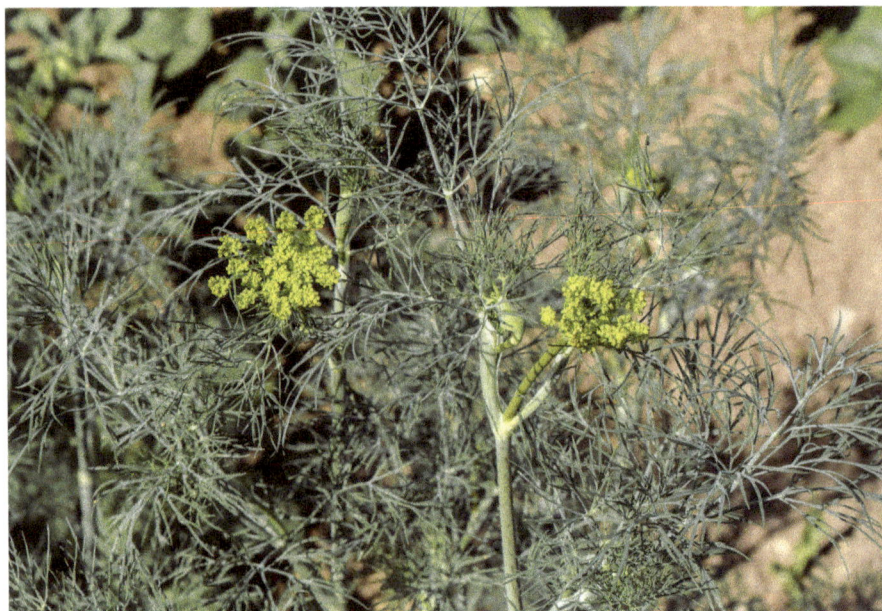

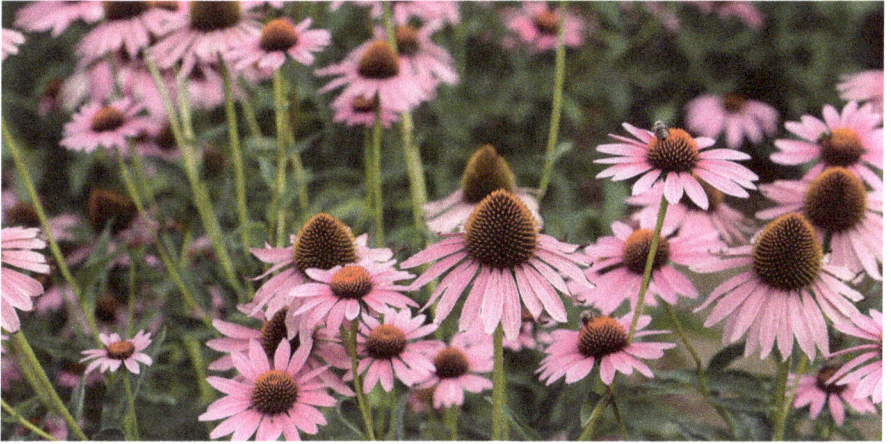

Echinacea

Echinacea purpurea
Perennial

Echinacea prefers full sun to partial shade. Sow seed in fertile, well-drained soil during early summer. Space plants two feet apart. Echinacea becomes dormant in the winter and re-emerges in the spring.

Garden Splendor: Sometimes known as purple coneflower, Echinacea produces rosy purple blooms.

Parts used: Roots are used medicinally. Leaves and flowers are edible.

To harvest: If using the roots for herbal remedies, the plant should be 3-4 years old. Dig up the roots when the plant dies back. Scrub. Use fresh or dry.

To use: Echinacea can help stimulate the immune system. It has antiviral and antibacterial properties. Fight cold and flu symptoms with Echinacea tea made from dried, fresh or powdered root.

Caution: Echinacea interacts with several drugs. Check with your doctor before medicinal use if taking other medications. Also, do not take if you have allergies or asthma. There have also been some side effects reported, such as headache, dizziness, nausea, constipation, mild stomach pain and skin rashes. Taking Echinacea longer than 8-10 weeks may weaken the immune system.

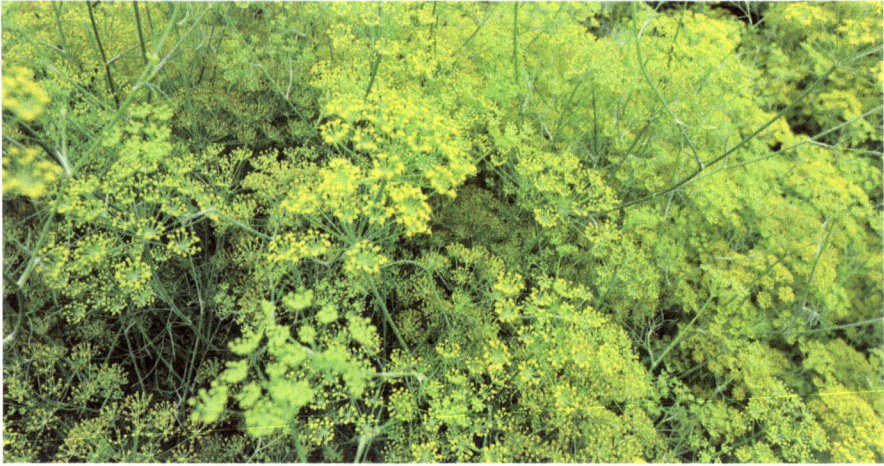

Fennel

Foeniculum vulgare
Perennial
Zones 6-9

Sow seeds in the garden in moderately fertile, well-drained soil. Fennel prefers full sun but tolerates partial shade. Space plants six inches apart. Fennel is short lived and often grown as an annual. Though it may not survive the winter, the seeds will produce new plants if allowed to drop.

Garden Splendor: Umbels of small yellow flowers appear above delicate, lacy leaves resembling dill.

Parts used: Leaves, stems and seeds

To harvest: Cut whole stems before the plant blooms, or collect the seedhead when seeds have dried and turned brown.

To use: The flavor of fennel is mild licorice. Use leaves in salads or other dishes. Eat stems the same way as celery. Seeds can be used whole or ground to flavor desserts. A fennel infusion aids digestion.

Caution: Fennel in medicinal amounts seems to affect estrogen levels in the body. Fennel may decrease the effects of birth control pills or estrogen pills.

Feverfew

Chrysanthemum parthenium
Perennial
Zones 5-7

Feverfew grows in full sun to partial shade in well-drained soil. Sow seed indoors in early spring. Space plants eighteen inches apart. Watch out for aphids. The plant is tough, but it can also be susceptible to root rot. Feverfew will also reseed prolifically, though individual plants usually die in their second or third summer. Feverfew can overwinter indoors.

Garden Splendor: Feverfew is in the daisy family. It has ferny leaves and small white flowers that bloom from midsummer to early fall. Bees do not like the odor of feverfew pollen, so they will not pollinate the nearby flowers that may be blooming at the same time.

Parts used: Leaves

To harvest: Cut leaves as needed.

To use: Feverfew does not help with fevers, but it can help prevent migraine headaches. Create an infusion or chew two fresh or frozen leaves regularly, gradually leading to less severe migraine headaches. Some people use it for arthritis and allergies, though studies do not support this.

Caution: Feverfew may cause a problem with blood clotting. Do not use medicinally if you have a heart disease or blood disorders, or you are taking aspirin. The leaves can also irritate the mouth. If this happens, discontinue use. Post-feverfew withdrawal syndrome can occur after using the herb for a long period of time. Symptoms include muscle stiffness, anxiety, headaches, and nausea. Do not use if you are allergic to ragweed, chrysanthemums, marigolds or related plants. Speak with your doctor before medicinal use if you are taking any other medications.

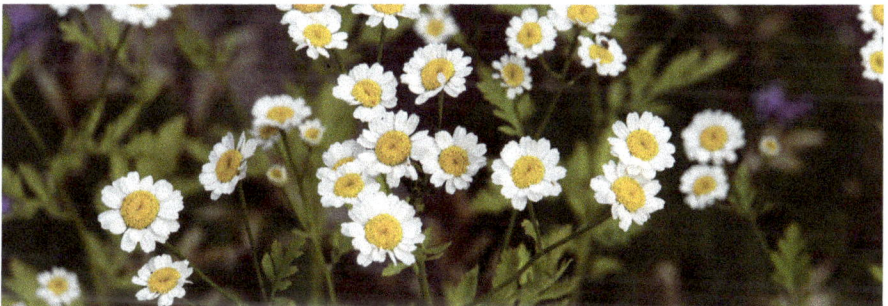

Garlic

Allium sativum
Perennial

Grow in full sun to light shade in deep, rich, well-drained soil. Plant individual cloves two inches deep and six inches apart in the mid-fall or early spring. If planting in fall, mulch for winter protection. Remove any flower stalks that form so that the plant will focus on growing the bulb rather than the flower.

Parts used: Leaves and cloves

To harvest: Dig up bulbs in late summer when tops die down and turn brown. Do not wash. Cure bulbs for 3-4 weeks by letting them dry in a cool, well-ventilated place away from sunlight. Store in a cool, dry place.

To use: Add garlic cloves to the many dishes that call for them. The green leaves can be also added to dishes and salads. For skin infections, apply a crushed garlic, garlic juice or infused garlic oil poultice. Fresh garlic is said to reduce cholesterol and blood pressure.

Caution: Though it is believed garlic can help with blood pressure and even treating cold symptoms, garlic can thin the blood. This increases the risk of bleeding, especially if taking blood-thinning medications for heart problems. Garlic is considered safe in amounts normally found in food, but it is possibly unsafe in medicinal amounts, such as garlic pills.

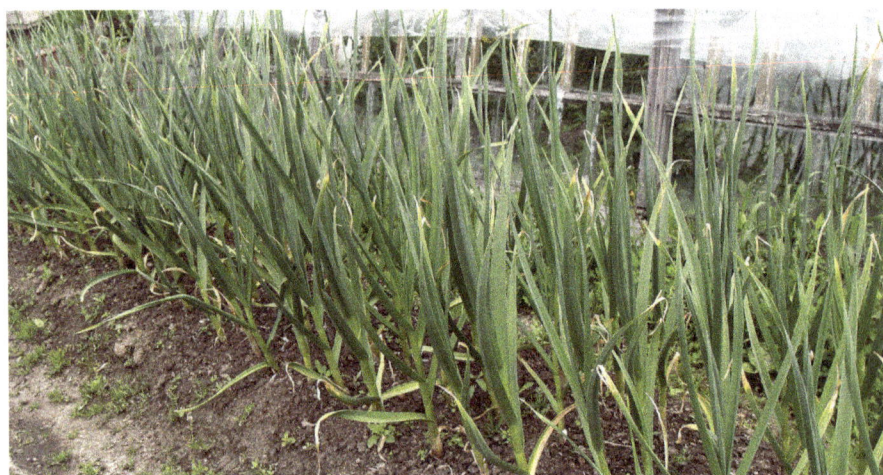

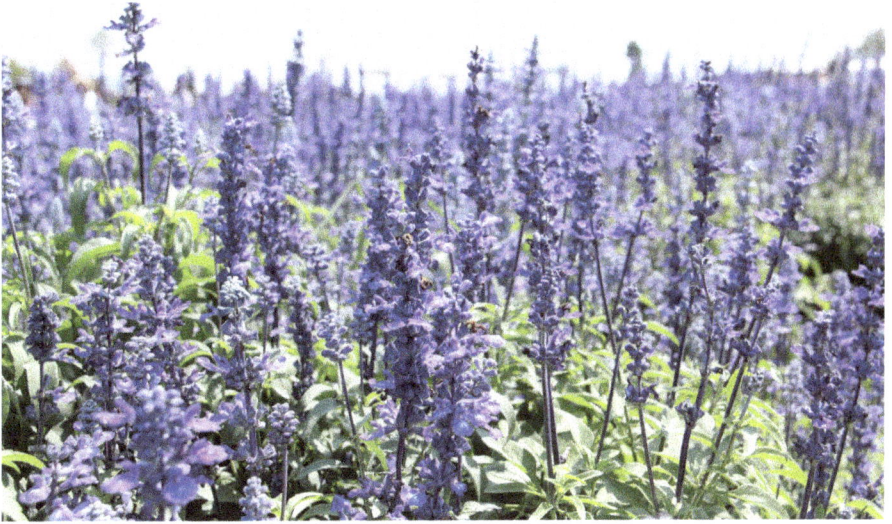

Hyssop

Hyssopus officinalis
Perennial
Zones 4-9

Hyssop prefers full sun but tolerates partial shade. Start with a plant or sow seed ¼-inch deep in well-drained, sandy soil. Set plants twelve inches apart. Hyssop is usually pest free but can be susceptible to root rot in poorly-drained soil.

Garden Splendor: Hyssop is topped with spikes of tiny blue or purple flowers.

Parts used: Flowers and leaves

To harvest: Snip portions of the stalk as needed, or cut whole branches for drying.

To use: The flavor of hyssop's leaves is mint. Use in salads, soups, stews and poultry stuffing. A tea can be brewed to ease coughs and respiratory irritation. The flavor becomes bitter if used in large quantities.

Caution: The oil product of hyssop may cause seizures in some people. It is especially not safe for children.

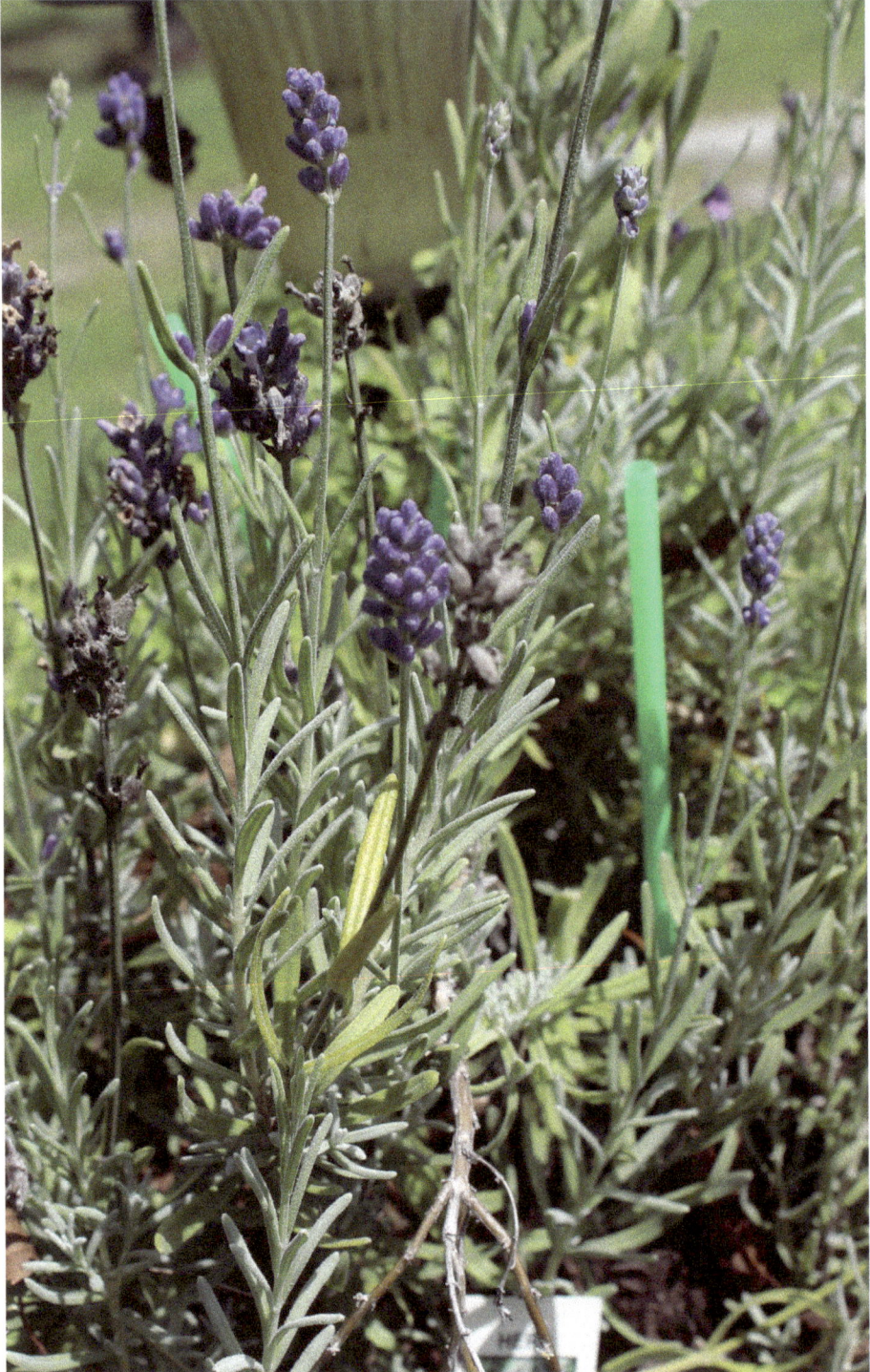

Lavender

Lavandula spp.
Perennial
Zones 5-8

Start seeds indoors 8-10 weeks before the last frost. Lavender prefers full sun but can grow in partial shade. It requires well-drained, moderately fertile soil. Space plants 1-3 feet apart. Lavender is generally pest-free. Leaf spot or root rot can develop. Pick off any infected leaves and prune to promote air circulation. Let soil dry between watering. Lavender will survive winter temperatures down to 0°F.

Garden Splendor: Lavender is aromatic. Each spike can grow to up to 1-3 feet. Depending on the species, the spikes are adorned with purple, pink, blue or white flowers.

Parts used: Leaves and flowers

To harvest: Cut flowers several inches below the bloom.

To use: Fresh springs can scent closets and drawers. Dried flowers are used for infusions. They can also be added to baked dishes, teas and jellies. Leaves are used in cooking. Lavender is also used in skin products or to scent oils and soaps. The most common species of lavender for medicinal use is *Lavandula angustifolia*. Lavender-infused oil helps to relieve pain from a burn. A cold compress of lavender may ease a headache. Lavender is also used to calm anxiety.

Caution: One side effect of lavender is sensitivity to sunlight. Though lavender is well tolerated, it may have weak hormonal effects. For example, excessive breast development was reported in preteen boys with repeated application of lavender and tea tree oils. Therefore, do not use if you have a hormone-sensitive cancer. Do not use if you are taking sedatives or hypnotic drugs, depressants, anticonvulsants or cholesterol-lowering drugs.

The abbreviation "spp." following the binomial species name refers to the group of species.

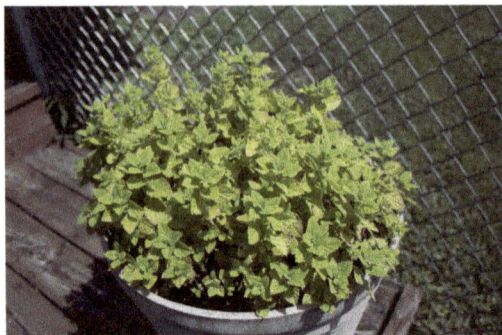

> ***Filtered Sun* refers to the sun shining on a plant through the leaves of another plant or a structure.**

Lemon Balm

Melissa officinalis
Perennial
Zones 4-9

Lemon balm prefers full sun in northern regions and filtered sun in the south. Space plants two feet apart in well-drained, average soil. Lemon balm is usually pest free. The plant is a mint, but it is not as invasive as other mints in the family. Lemon balm can survive winter temperatures to -20°F.

Garden Splendor: Lemon balm has a lemon flavor and fragrance.

Parts used: Leaves

To harvest: Snip stems at leaf nodes for a sprig of leaves as needed.

To use: Used for flavoring in salads, sauces and many dishes. Lemon balm is also used in herbal teas. Medicinally, lemon balm is possibly effective for anxiety. Some studies have shown that lotions with lemon balm can reduce agitation in people with dementia. Lip balm made with lemon balm extract can reduce symptoms of recurring cold sore infections on the mouth.

Caution: Do not take lemon balm medicinally if you have a thyroid disease, diabetes or upcoming surgery. Lemon balm causes drowsiness. Do not take with other sedatives. Other side effects can also occur.

Note: Other lemony garden herbs to try are Lemongrass (Cymbopogon citratus) and Lemon verbena (Aloysia triphylla).

Marjoram

Origanum majorana
Tender perennial
Zones 9-10

Sweet marjoram is usually grown as an annual. It prefers full sun but tolerates partial shade. Soil should be rich and well-drained. If planting seeds, sow indoors and leave uncovered. In the garden, space clumps of plants eight inches apart. Marjoram is usually pest and disease free. The plant remains hardy only in mild winters. In cold climates, overwinter indoors.

Garden Splendor: Marjoram is a sweeter version of oregano. It has a mild aroma and is topped with tiny blooms.

Parts used: Leaves

To harvest: Harvest leaves as needed. Before flowers bloom, cut whole stems for drying.

To use: Use leaves and flowers in dishes and salads the same way oregano is used. Sweet marjoram tea may soothe an upset stomach.

Caution: Used medicinally for long term, marjoram may have serious side effects, such as damage to liver and kidneys. Medicinal amounts may also slow blood clotting. Those with bleeding disorders or an upcoming surgery should avoid marjoram.

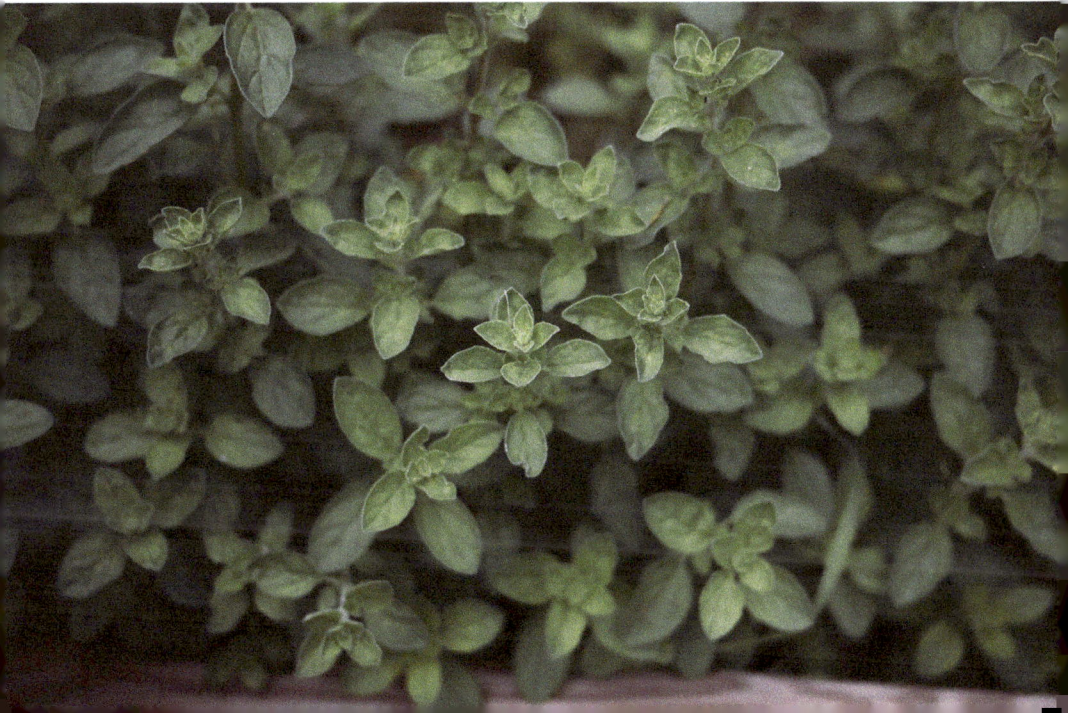

Mints

Mentha spp.
Perennial
Zones 5-9

   Mints are not usually true-to-seed and should be purchased from the nursery. Mint plants grow in full sun to partial shade in rich, moist well-drained soil. Place plants in the garden eighteen inches apart or in a large container. Most of these aromatic species are deemed invasive with their spreading roots. They will also self-seed. Mint is hardy even in cold climates. The plants have some pest enemies, such as aphids, spider mites, mint flea beetles and cutworms. They can also be susceptible to some diseases.

Parts used: Leaves

To harvest: Pick leaves as needed, or cut whole stems to within a few inches of the ground. Cut plants to the ground after the last harvest. After flowers have formed and gone to seed, the taste of the leaves is believed to change.

To use: Use leaves in dishes, candies, jellies, sauces, teas, and more. Mints have a reputation of helping ease indigestion and relieving congestion. Peppermint tea is a possible stomach soother. Topically, due to menthol, the peppermint species (*Mentha piperita*) can also relive pain and itching.

Caution: Speak with your doctor before medicinal use if you are taking other medications. Peppermint essential oil has additional cautions, including risk of toxicity.

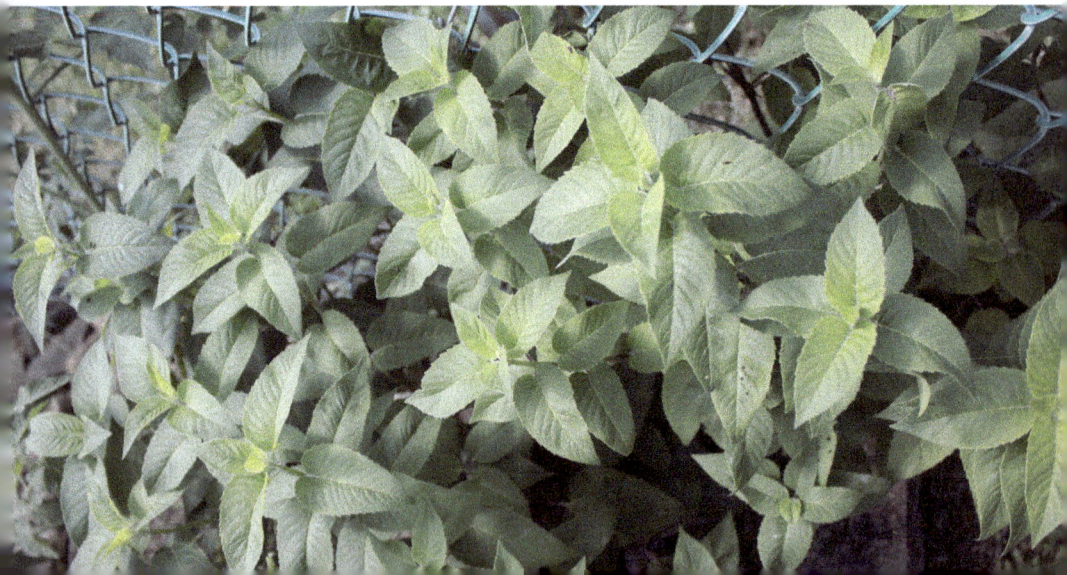

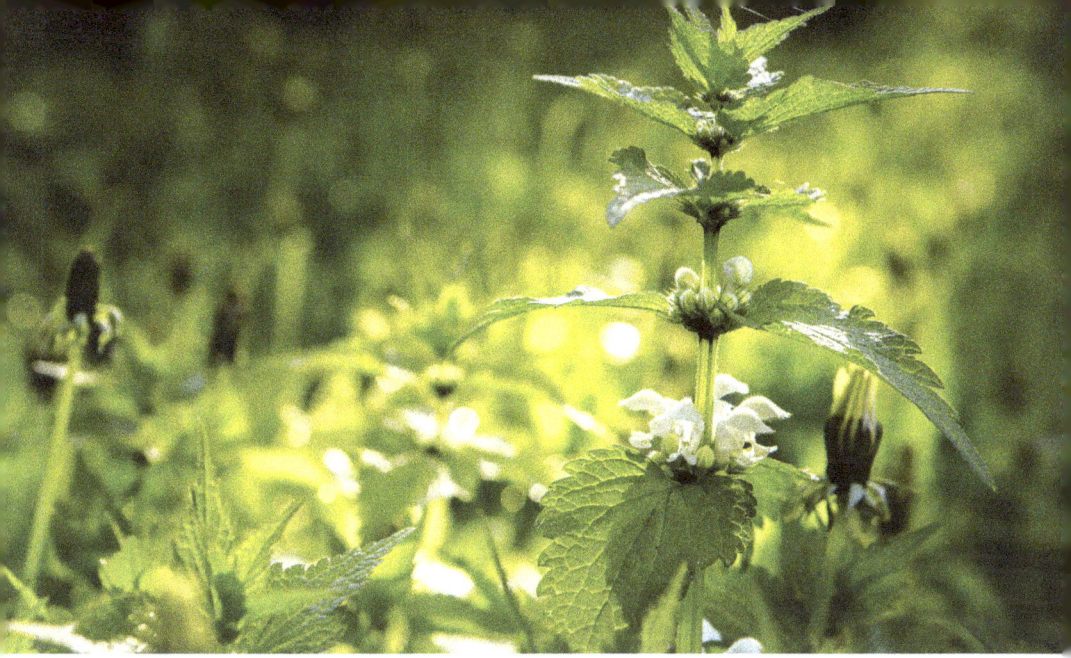

Nettle

Urtica dioica
Tender perennial

Stinging nettle flourishes in temperate climates of many parts of the world. Not all plants of the species sting, but this plant of the Urticaceae family is most known for causing a stinging sensation to the skin. You are probably already familiar with nettle growing up unwanted in your garden.

Parts used: Leaves

To harvest: Use gloves unless harvesting young nettle.

To use: The sting of nettle can be eliminated quickly by cooking it. Cooked leaves may be added to culinary dishes. Nettle has also been shown to treat urinary tract disorders. Clinical trials support topical use of nettle for arthritis. The plant is believed to treat other conditions, including allergies and inflammation. However, proper evidence is still lacking.

Caution: Several medications interact with nettle. Touching the plant may cause skin irritation.

Oregano

Origanum heracleoticum
Perennial
Zones 5-9

This aromatic herb needs full sun and average, well-drained soil. Space plants eight inches apart. Established plants will self-seed. They are very vivacious. Aphids, leafminers and spider mites are pests of oregano. Plants can also contract root rot or leaf spot. Oregano stays hardy through the winter of cold climates if well rooted and mulched.

Parts used: Leaves

To harvest: Snip sprigs as needed when the plant is at least six inches high. Before the flower buds, cut all stems to within an inch of the ground.

To use: Add leaves to tomato dishes or many other meals. Oregano can make very flavorful infused oil. Oregano tea settles the stomach or soothes a cough. It may also help with digestion. Oregano has been touted to fight against bacteria, viruses, funguses and parasites.

Caution: Oregano may increase the risk of bleeding in people with bleeding disorders. For the same reason, if scheduled for a surgery, discontinue use a few weeks prior. Those with diabetes should use oregano with caution as it may lower blood sugar levels. Speak with your doctor before medicinal use if you are taking other medications.

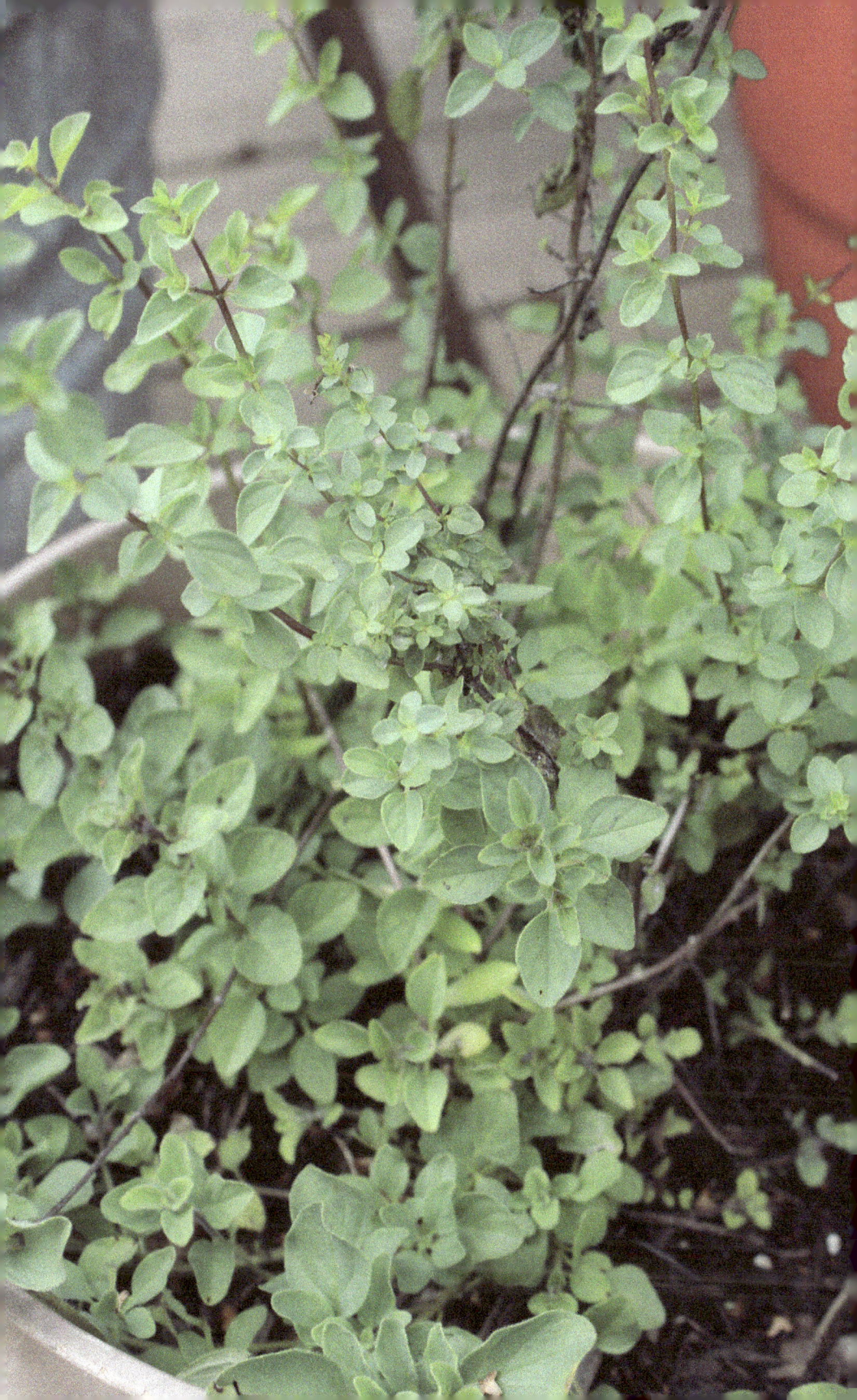

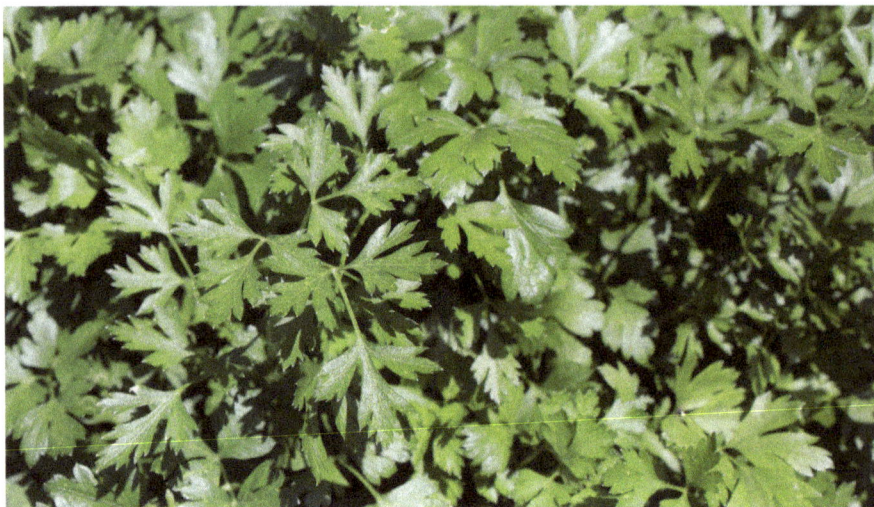

Parsley

Petroselinum crispum
Biennial
Zones 5-9

Parsley is fragrant and easy to grow. In the second year, it will produce flowers that attract beneficial insects. Parsley grows in full sun or partial shade with moderately rich, moist well-drained soil. Thin seedlings to stand eight inches apart. Pot parsley in early fall and bring inside to grow through the winter. Parsley is hardy to 10°F.

Parts used: Leaves

To harvest: Cut stems one inch above the crown of the plant. Pruning promotes leaf production.

To use: Add to dishes and salads. Parsley's high chlorophyll content makes it a natural breath freshener. Chew some fresh sprigs for the effect. Parsley can help prevent dandruff when added to a hair conditioner. Parsley tea may help relieve hay fever and hives.

Caution: Parsley in medicinal amounts can interact with some drugs and affect some chronic conditions. It also causes photosensitivity.

Rosemary

Rosmarinus officinalis
Tender perennial
Zones 8-10

Rosemary does well in full sun and well-drained soil. Space plants 12-18 inches apart. In a cooler zone, grow in a large, deep container and bring indoors for the winter. Watch out for some pests like mealybugs and whiteflies. Root rot and botrytis blight can also affect this plant. Rosemary is hardy in winter to 10°F.

Parts used: Flowers and leaves

To harvest: Cut rosemary shoot tips as needed. Flowers can be picked and used also.

To use: Use leaves and flowers for garnishing food and flavoring oils. Crush or mince leaves before adding to dishes. Rosemary tea has been said to soothe digestive upsets and relieve menstrual cramping. Taking rosemary may improve memory and alertness.

Caution: Those with an aspirin allergy, bleeding disorder or seizure disorder should not use rosemary medicinally.

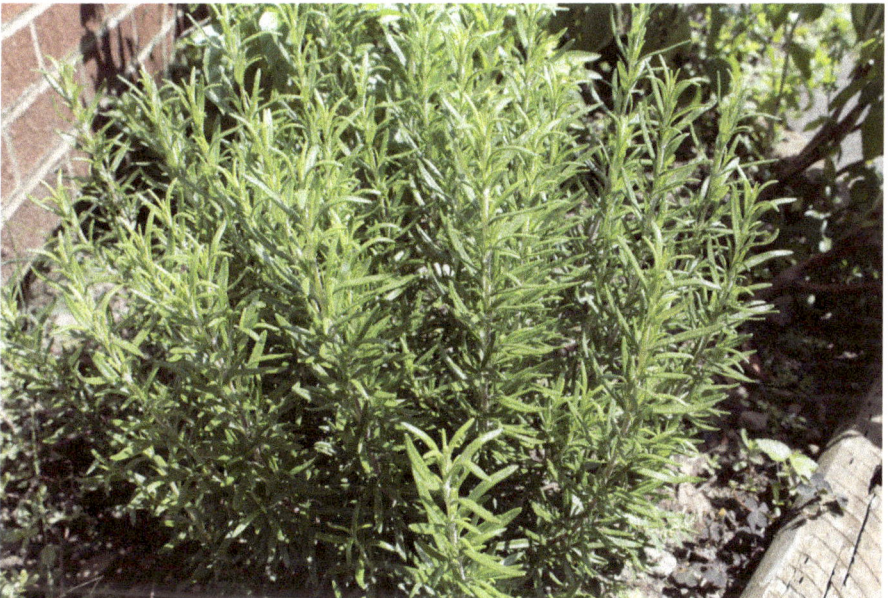

Saffron

Crocus sativus
Perennial
Zones 6-9

Plant saffron corms root-side down a few inches into well-drained soil of average fertility. Space corms six inches apart. Saffron prefers partial shade but tolerates full sun. Plants are pest free but can be susceptible to root rot in poorly drained soil.

Garden Splendor: Plants produce purple crocus flowers with yellow stigmas.

Parts used: Stigmas

To harvest: Harvest stigmas when flowers are fully open in the morning and before insects begin pollinating them.

To use: Saffron has a lightly bitter taste. The fragrance is spicy and pungent. Stigmas are used in cooking, though it takes several plants to grow the quantity needed for recipes. Saffron extract may reduce depression symptoms.

Caution: High doses of saffron can cause poisoning. Saffron seems to lower blood pressure and affect moods. Those with bipolar disorder or heart conditions should avoid saffron in medicinal doses.

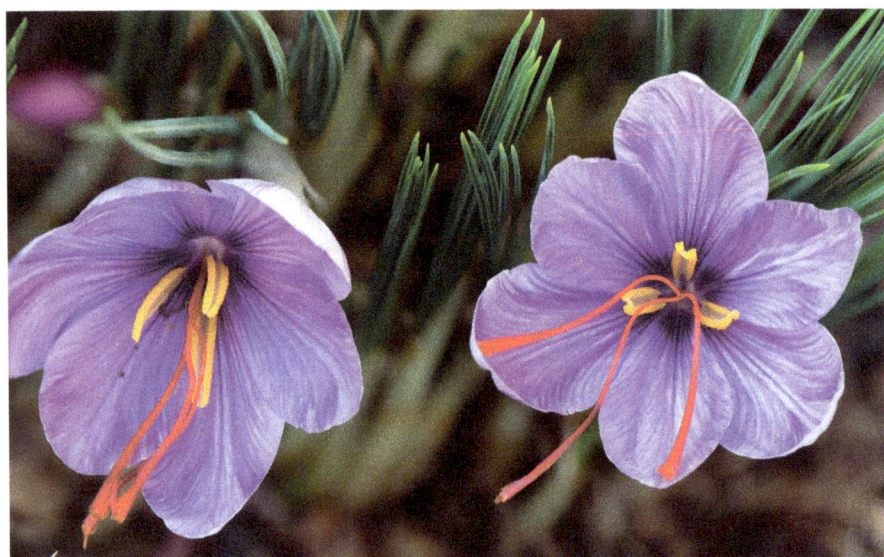

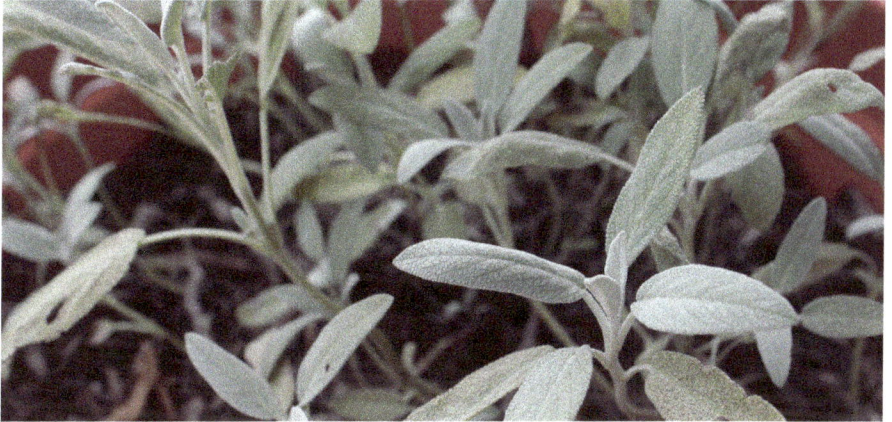

Sage

Salvia officinalis
Perennial
Zones 4-8

Sage grows best in full sun and well-drained, moderately rich soil. Space transplants or thin seedlings about twenty inches apart. Pests can be spider mites, spittlebugs and slugs. The plant is susceptible to some diseases. Sage is hardy in winter to 15°F. It can be potted and overwintered inside.

Garden Splendor: Sage's bright pink, purple, blue or white flowers grow in whorls. Plants stand as tall as three feet.

Parts used: Leaves

To harvest: Pick leaves as needed or harvest whole stems before the flower buds.

To use: This aromatic herb can flavor oils and add fragrance to stuffings, breads and many dishes. Infusions are said to soothe sore throats, tone the skin and deodorize. Sage extracts can possibly improve mental performance.

Caution: Taking common sage medicinally for long term may be toxic or cause seizures. Sage may also act like estrogen in the body. It interacts with some medications, such as diabetes medications.

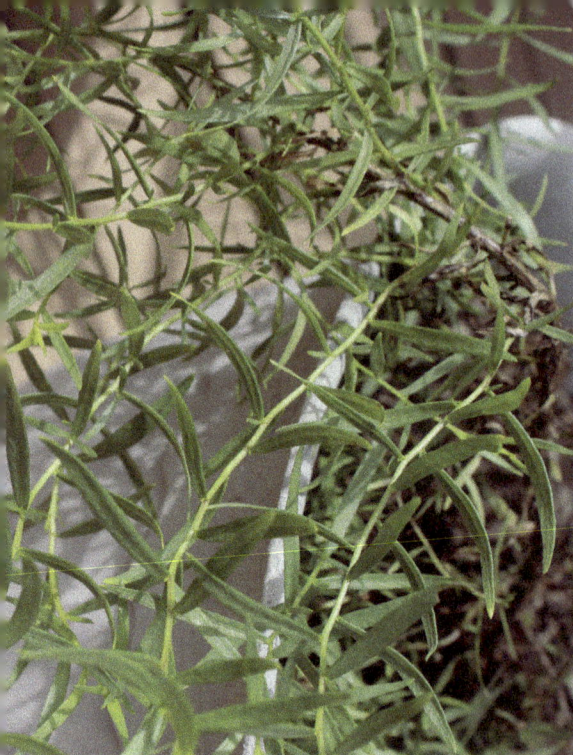

Tarragon, French

Artemisia dracunculus var. sativa
Perennial
Zones 4-8

Note that the Russian tarragon lacks the aromatic oils of the French tarragon. French tarragon grows in full sun to partial shade in rich, well-drained soil. Space plants two feet apart. Mulch in the winter to protect from frost. Roots can be divided every few years to help keep plants vigorous. Tarragon can survive in winter to -20°F.

Parts used: Leaves

To harvest: Harvest branch tips as needed in early summer. Cut back to stimulate new growth. Dried tarragon loses its oil. Preserve by freezing or storing in white vinegar.

To use: The licorice flavor of tarragon is quite strong. Make a tarragon vinegar or use in many recipes. Heal herpes outbreaks with a tarragon and lemon balm tea. Relieve minor mouth pain temporarily by chewing tarragon leaves.

Caution: Long-term use of tarragon as a medicine may be unsafe. Tarragon may also slow blood clotting. Those with bleeding disorders or upcoming surgery should use caution if using tarragon medicinally.

The abbreviation "var." indicates the variety.

118

Thyme

Thymus spp.
Perennial
Zones 5-9

This shrubby, aromatic herb grows well in full sun and light, dry, well-drained soil. Transplant seedlings twelve inches apart. Replace plants every two or three years as they become woody. Watch out for spider mites, root rot and leaf spot. Thyme becomes dormant in the winter and re-emerges in the spring.

Parts used: Leaves

To harvest: Pick sprigs as needed. The whole plant can be harvested by cutting it down to two inches from the ground.

To use: Thyme is used to season many French foods. It has antibacterial and antifungal activity and can relieve coughs. Brew a tea to calm a cough or soothe the stomach.

Caution: Used medicinally, thyme might act like estrogen in the body. It may also slow blood clotting. Those with hormone sensitive conditions, bleeding disorders or upcoming surgery should use caution.

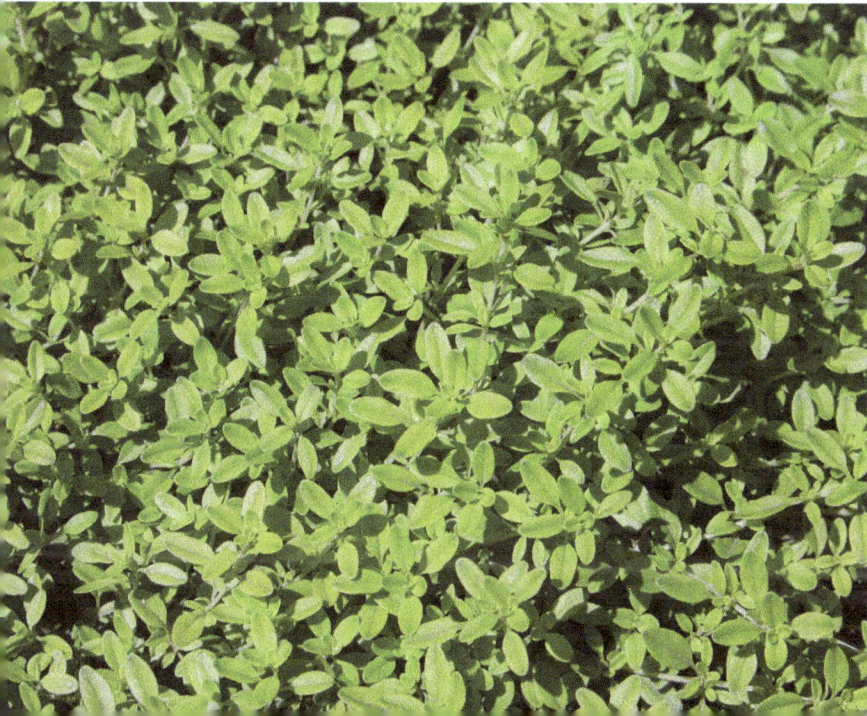

119

Valerian

Valeriana officinalis
Perennial

Grow in full sun to partial shade in rich, moist soil. Set plants twelve inches apart. Valerian should be divided regularly. It may be necessary to protect the plants from cats. It is usually pest and disease free. Valerian dies back to the ground in winter and re-emerges in the spring.

Garden Splendor: This is a spreading herb with large clusters of small pink or white flowers. It can grow to five feet tall.

Parts used: Roots

To harvest: Harvest roots in fall or spring before new shoots appear. Wash and dry in an oven until brittle. Store in an airtight container.

To use: Valerian is used to improve sleep and help with anxiety over time. Make a calming tea with two teaspoons of powdered root per one cup of water. Sweeteners will be needed because the taste is bitter. Add to bathwater for a calming soak.

Caution: Valerian contains a potent active ingredient that causes sedation. Use only for a limited period of time. Extended use can cause depression. Valerian should never be given to children. Valerian products might also interact with a number of drugs or health conditions. Speak with your doctor before medicinal use.

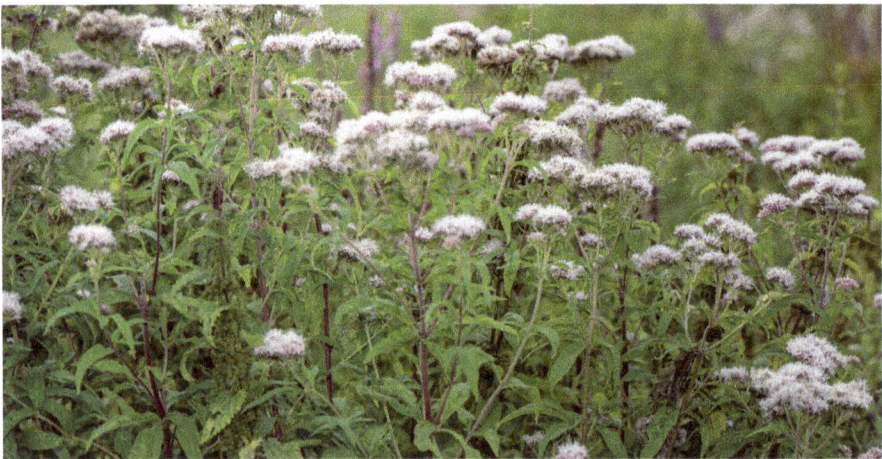

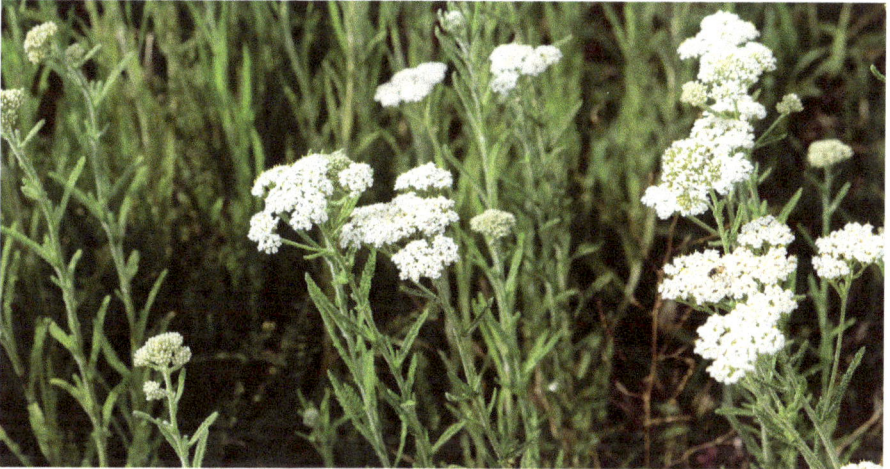

Yarrow

Achillea millefolium
Perennial
Zones 4-7

Yarrow has come to the United States from Europe. The plant grows well in full sun and moderately rich, well-drained soil. Set plants or thin seedlings twelve inches apart. Divide the plants every few years. Yarrow can spread by runners. Pull out unwanted growths. Yarrow may suffer from a few diseases, such as powdery mildew or stem rot. It is usually pest free. Cut back plants to within six inches of the ground after flowering to prepare for winter.

Garden Splendor: Clusters of bright flowers attract beneficial insects, including tiny wasps that feed on aphids.

Parts used: Leaves

To harvest: Pick leaves as needed or harvest the whole plant by cutting to one inch above the ground as the flowers come to bloom.

To use: Yarrow is used to treat minor wounds, aid digestion and relieve menstrual cramps. It can be added to skin lotions as an astringent. In a hair conditioner, it tempers oily hair. Make a soothing tea with added sweeteners to taste. Apply an unsweetened infusion to wounds and inflammations.

Caution: Beware of allergic reactions if taking internally. Yarrow might slow blood clotting. Those with bleeding disorders or upcoming surgery should not use.

A Parting Word

Herbs allow us to add more flavor to our meals, save money on household products and have a natural first aid kit at our fingertips. Weeds are not so ugly and bothersome as we learn more about the plants that surround us.

But thinking about many herbs can be overwhelming. How will we ever learn it all? Not to mention that there are several dangers in plant medicine.

Don't worry. For all of history, people primarily had access only to indigenous, local herbs, not hundreds of herbs from all over the world like we do today. Working with just a few herbs safely can be enough to enrich your life the ways you were hoping when you first picked up this book.

In the meantime, I trust that the information provided in these pages has brought to light realities of both Herbal Medicine and herbalism. Along this journey, you will meet the sweet Kathys of the world who pass down timeless gardening wisdom and treasured recipes. But you will also encounter individuals who have been deceived in some way. They will share what they have learned, too. The realm of plant medicine is an area for Christians to be vigilant, bold and uncompromising. We do not have to live in fear, but we are commanded to be set apart.

Most of my own experience with occult deception in herbalism occurred in the subfield of aromatherapy. Although I would not consider myself an expert herb crafter, the text for this book was reviewed by experienced gardeners as well as other Bible teachers. I wrote it because I felt that books like this one could not be available soon enough.

In the end, I pray that *The Christian Herb Gardener's Handbook* has been a blessing to you, dear brothers and sisters.

Peace to you in Christ Jesus,

Meg Grimm

Special Thanks

My friend Marci Julin - for her wise guidance, support and help with editing.

My sister-in-law Jessica Thompson and my husband Max Grimm –
for providing most of the dazzling photography for this book.

My friend Kathy Bota – for the use of her beautiful yard for photos, and for
sharing her gardening tips and special recipes.

My writing group pals, Kristy Clements and Gwen Shimko -
for their suggestions and encouragement.

How to Become a Christian

The Bible teaches that all have sinned and deserve God's judgment. But God so loved the world that He sent His only Son Jesus, who lived a sinless life and died in our place.

Jesus took our punishment instead! He resurrected from the dead three days later, defeating sin and death forever. If you believe this, repent of your sin and choose to trust Jesus, declaring that He is Lord and God. You will be saved from judgment and live eternally with Him in heaven. (John 1:12, 3:16.)

As a Christian (Christ follower), seek to become involved in a Bible-believing church fellowship. This is God's design for strengthening your own faith as well as blessing other believers, who are now your brothers and sisters in God's family. (Heb.10:24-25) Align yourself with Christian mentors who will help you understand all that took place at the moment of your salvation in Christ and who will walk with you on the next steps on this journey. Regularly read your Bible and pray to deepen in your personal relationship with Jesus. (Ps. 1:1-2, 1 Thess. 5:16-18)

Jesus loves you and has been waiting for you! He has a plan and purpose for your life, more than all you could ask for or imagine. (Eph. 3:14-21)

Recommended Resources

Christian Resources on Alternative Medicine Therapies

Alternative Medicine: The Christian Handbook

O'Mathúna, Dónal and Walt Larimore. Grand Rapids, Mich.:
    Zondervan, 2007. Print.
    *The claims and the evidence from a Christian perspective, with two
    references sections: 1) Alternative therapies, and 2) Herbal remedies,
    vitamins and dietary supplements.*

Can You Trust Your Doctor: The Complete Guide to New Age Medicine and Its Threat to Your Family

Ankerberg, John and Weldon, John. Brentwood, Tenn: Wolgemutch
    & Hyatt, Publishers, Inc. 1991. Print.
    *A comprehensive list of New Age medicine techniques, offering knowl-
    edge and information needed for wise decisions.*

Biblical Medicine

Life to the Body: Biblical Principles for Health & Healing

Julin, Marci. 2019. Print.
    *Where do we turn when alternative medicine becomes spiritually dan-
    gerous but conventional medicine disappoints? These are not our only
    two options. Christian speaker and author Marci Julin reveals a Biblical
    model for healthcare.*

Herbals

Tyler's Honest Herbal: A Sensible Guide to the Use of Herbs and Related Remedies (4th edition)

Foster, Steven, and Varro E. Tyler. London: Haworth Press, 1999. Print.

Herbs of the Bible: 2000 Years of Plant Medicine

Duke, James A. Loveland, Col.: Interweave Press, 1999. Print.

Wildcrafting Field Guide

Newcomb's Wildflower Guide
Newcomb, Lawrence. Little, Brown and Company, 1977. Print.

Herbal Monograph Databases

Pharmacist's Letter/Natural Medicines Comprehensive Database
Jellin, Jeff M., Forrest Batz, and Kathy Hichens. Stockton, Calif:
Therapeutic Research Facility, 1999. Print.
Also available by subscription online at www.naturaldatabase.com

U.S. National Library of Medicine: MedlinePlus Herbs and Supplements
https://medlineplus.gov/druginfo/herb_All.html

National Center for Complementary and Integrative Health: Herbs at a Glance
https://nccih.nih.gov/health/herbsataglance.htm

Memorial Sloan Kettering Cancer Center: About Herbs, Botanicals and Other Products
https://www.mskcc.org/cancer-care/diagnosis-treatment/symp
tommanagement/integrative-medicine/herbs

Professional's Handbook of Complementary and Alternative Medicine
Fetrow, Charles W., and Juan R. Avila. Springhouse, Pa.: Sprinhouse, 2001.
Print.

Other Databases

U.S. Food and Drug Poisonous Plant Database
https://www.cfsanappsexternal.fda.gov/scripts/plantox/index.cfm

National Institutes of Health, PubMed Dietary Supplement Subset
https://ods.od.nih.gov/Research/PubMed_Dietary_Supplement_
Subset. aspx

Herb Gardening

The Best Little Herb Book
Defalco, Josephine. Flint Hills Publishing: Topeka, Kans. 2017. Print.

Your Backyard Herb Garden
Smith, Miranda. Emmaus, Pa.: Rodale Press, Inc. 1997. Print.

Vegetable & Herb Gardening

Grow What You Eat, Eat What You Grow
Shore, Randy. Vancouver, Canada: Arsenal Pulp Press, 2014. Print.

Identifying Pests

Dr. Bader's Pest Cures: Natural Solutions to Things That Bug You!
Bader, Myles. Fairfield, NJ: TeleBrands Press. 2012. Print.

Soapmaking

Simple & Natural Soapmaking
Berry, Jan. Salem, Mass.: Page Street Publishing Co. 2017. Print.

The Natural Soapmaking Book for Beginners
Cable, Kelly. Berkeley, CA: Althea Press. 2017. Print.

Crafting Teas

Tea for You
Stern, Tracy. New York: Clarkson Potter/Publishers. 2009. Print.

Works Consulted & Notes

Reference notes in this book refer to a number for a title listed below followed by page numbers, if applicable. For example, 18:203 would refer to page 203 of Alternative Medicine: The Christian Handbook.

1) Ankerberg, John and John Weldon. *Can You Trust Your Doctor: The Complete Guide to New Age Medicine and Its Threat to Your Family.* (1st edition). Wolgemutch & Hyatt, Publishers, Inc., Brentwood, Tennessee. 1991. Print.

2) Berry, Jan. *Simple & Natural Soapmaking.* Salem, Ma: Page Street Publishing Co. 2017. Print.

3) Cook, Michelle Schoffro. *Be Your Own Herbalist.* Canada: New World Library. 2016. Print.

4) Davey, Melissa. "Herbal medicines can have dangerous side effects, research reveals." The Guardian, 5 Feb 2017. Accessed 2019 through www.theguardian.com/australia-news/2017/feb/06/herbal-medicines-can-have-dangerous-side-effects-research-reveals

5) Duke, James A. *Herbs of the Bible: 2000 Years of Plant Medicine.* Loveland, Col.: Interweave Press, 1999. Print.

6) Earle, Liz. *Skin Care Secrets.* Buffalo, New York: Firefly Books. 2010. Print.

7) Edgar, Julie. "Types of Teas and Their Health Benefits." WebMD, s.d. Accessed 25 Sept 2019 through https://www.webmd.com/diet/features/tea-types-and-their-health-benefits

8) Ecklund, Doug. "Herbalism: Medicine or Mysticism." (s.l., s.d.) Accessed 2019 through http://logosresourcepages.org/NewAge/herbalism.htm

9) N. "Herbal Supplements: Helpful or Harmful." Cleveland Clinic, s.d. Accessed 2019 through https://my.clevelandclinic.org/health/articles/17095

10) N. "Herbal Supplements You Shouldn't Try." WebMD, s.d. Accessed 2019 through www.webmd.com/vitamins-and-supplements/ss/slide-show-herbs-supplements-avoid

11) Kee, Howard Clark. *Medicine, Miracle and Magic in New Testament Times.* Cambridge, New York: Cambridge University Press. 1986. Print.

12) Lee, Elizabeth. "Beware of Sunburn Boosters." WebMD, s.d. Accessed 24 Sept 2019 through https://www.webmd.com/beware-of-sun burn-boosters

13) Newmaster, Steven G., Et. al. "DNA barcoding detects contamination and substitution in North American herbal products." 2013. BMC Medicine, 1 (11) pp. 222. Accessed 2019 through https://doi.org/10.1186/1741-7015-11-222

14) Memorial Sloan Kettering Cancer Center: About Herbs, Botanicals and Other Products, Herbal Monographs URL: https://www.mskcc.org/cancer-care/diagnosis-treatment/symp-tom-management/integrative-medicine/herbs

15) MedlinePlus Herbs and Supplements, Herbal Monographs (U.S. National Library of Medicine) URL: https://medlineplus.gov/druginfo/herb_All.html

16) Millunchick, Mordechai. "Ahala, Boris – Soap." Trees in the Daf, s.d. Accessed 25 Sept 2019 through https://treesinthedaf.word press.com/2017/08/29/ahala

17) O'Connor, Anahad. "Herbal Supplements are Often not What They Seem." New York Times. 3 Nov 2013. Accessed 2019 through https://nyti.ms/1bQ9QbC

18) O'Mathúna, Dónal and Walt Larimore. *Alternative Medicine: The Christian Handbook (Updated Expanded).* Zondervan, Grand Rapids, Michigan. 2007. Print.

19) N. "Photodermatitis." Penn State Hershey, Milton S. Hershey Medical Center, s.d. Accessed 25 Sept 2019 through http://pennstatehershey.adam.com/content.aspx?productId=107&pid=33&gid=000155

20) Preuss, Julius (1911). *Biblical and Talmudic Medicine*. Translated by Dr. Fred Rosner, Northvale, New Jersey: Jason Aronson Inc., 1993. Print.

21) Smith, Miranda. *Your Backyard Herb Garden*. Emmaus, Pa: Rodale Press, Inc. 1997. Print.

22) *The A-Z Guide to Herbs That Heal*. Emmaus, Pa: Rodale Press, Inc. 1995. Print.

23) Stern, Tracy. *Tea for You*. New York: Clarkson Potter/Publishers. 2009. Print.

24) Timberlake, Sean. "What is Pectin in Jams and Jellies?" The Spruce Eats, 24 Mar 2019. Accessed 25 Sept 2019 through https://www.thespruceeats.com/what-is-pectin-1327810

25) University of Adelaide. "Herbal medicines can be lethal, pathologist warns." ScienceDaily. ScienceDaily, 12 February 2010. Accessed 29 Jan 2020 through www.sciencedaily.com/releases/2010/02/100209183337.htm

26) Vamosh, Miriam Feinberg. *Food at the Time of the Bible*. Herzlia, Israel: Palphot Ltd. (s.d.) Print.

27) Visser, Meagan. "What Every Herbalist Should Know About Herbal Preparation." The Herbal Academy, 27 Aug 2018. Accessed 12 Jan 2020 through https://theherbalacademy.com/herbal-preparation-shelf-life/

www.ingramcontent.com/pod-product-compliance
Lightning Source LLC
Chambersburg PA
CBHW041215030426
42336CB00023B/3352